conquering
EATING DISORDERS

HOW FAMILY COMMUNICATION HEALS

Sue Cooper, PhD and
Peggy Norton, RD

SEAL PRESS

Conquering Eating Disorders
How Family Communication Heals

Published by Seal Press
A Member of the Perseus Books Group
1700 Fourth Street
Berkeley, CA 94710

Library of Congress Cataloging-in-Publication Data
Cooper, Susan M.
  Conquering eating disorders : how family communication heals / by
Susan M. Cooper and Peggy Norton.
    p. cm.
  ISBN-13: 978-1-58005-260-3
  ISBN-10: 1-58005-260-6
  1. Eating disorders in adolescence--Popular works. 2. Eating
disorders in adolescence--Patients--Family relationships. I. Norton,
Peggy. II. Title.
  RJ506.E18C66 2008
  616.85'26--dc22
                              2008020837

Cover design by Gerilyn Attebery
Interior design by Tabitha Lahr
Printed in the United States of America
Distributed by Publishers Group West

DEDICATION

In loving memory of Rosemary Syverson, our dear friend
and colleague whose life touched so many. We miss her
wisdom, her wonderful sense of humor, and her friendship.

contents

INTRODUCTION

THE POWER OF LOVE

The most basic and powerful way to connect with another
person is to listen. Just listen. Perhaps the most important
thing we ever give each other is our attention. . . . A loving
silence often has far more power to heal and to connect than
the most well-intentioned words.

—Rachel Naomi Remen

An eating disorder creeps into a teenager's life like a parasite, draining away the precious life force of its victim. But instead of sensing the attack, the teen almost always perceives the eating disorder as a rescuer—whether it be from unpopularity, obesity, or feelings of being trapped, scared, angry, or lonely. On some level, the victim may know she's in trouble, and yet it seems unthinkable to betray the perceived rescuer. She often develops a strong loyalty toward her eating disorder—a reaction not unlike Stockholm syndrome, in which a hostage develops deep empathy with her captor. This tendency, coupled with the gradual and insidious nature of the attack, has surely contributed to the steady rise of eating disorders in Western society.

Women are not the only ones prone to eating disorders. Men are currently shown to represent 6 to 10 percent of individuals with eating disorders, but this percentage may be underreported because of the shame involved in having a disorder commonly associated with women.[1]

Disordered or dysfunctional eating is a growing problem as well, though not one serious enough to be classified as a clinical eating disorder. It is estimated that 40 to 50 percent of young women on college campuses struggle with body dissatisfaction and are currently restricting calories or engaging in various kinds of abnormal or inappropriate eating behaviors. High school girls report a constant preoccupation with weight concerns, and it is becoming more prevalent that children as young as four years old are eating only a small amount because they are afraid of being fat.[2] Young men also are increasingly at risk for disordered eating. The middle or high school wrestler who fasts for two days to make weight is a typical example. And the pressure on young men to meet the new ideal of a well-muscled or sculpted body is adding to this trend.

Eating disorders are, in essence, a cry for help. But since teens are only just beginning to find their voices, their cries for help rarely reach the volume of a blood-curdling scream. Usually the cry is a barely audible whimper—one that is all too easily drowned out in the chaos and clamor of today's world.

From time immemorial, coming of age has always been challenging, just by virtue of the fact that teenage bodies and social lives change so rapidly. But contemporary life offers many other challenges for today's teens and their parents. The constant barrage of media and advertising is rife with convincing messages that physical self-improvement is the key to love, success, and happiness. As a result, dieting has become a national obsession for many adults and teens, who seek status and admiration by trying to become unnaturally thin. Fashion magazines have contributed to the problem by filling their pages with anorexic and airbrushed models, who are then scrutinized and admired by impressionable teens. More and more, family structures are crumbling, leaving teens vulnerable to finding unhealthy ways of defining themselves and building self-esteem.

Surrounded by all of these challenges, parents and teens dealing with an eating disorder may feel as if they are on a battlefield. And in many ways, they are right.

THE PURPOSE OF THIS BOOK

We have written this book because we are on the front lines of this battle, and we see its casualties and its heroes on an ongoing basis. And we have seen, time and time again, that it is entirely possible for teens to emerge victorious, healthy, and free. The key, virtually every time, is honest, open communication—and this takes work, from everyone involved.

Our intentions are to shed light on how eating-disordered adolescents and their parents think, and to suggest ways for both parties to engage in open and affirming conversations that can avert the progression of an eating disorder, opening a path to recovery. In addition, we hope this book will enhance your awareness of what can trigger the development of an eating disorder. We also wish to challenge you to make changes in how you relate to one another, and to inspire you to seek the support you need for yourself and for those you care about.

It is *not* our intention to place blame, or to suggest that parents have caused the condition. The last thing we want is for anyone to get lost in guilt, as self-blame quickly becomes an exercise in self-absorption, diverting what should be a focus on recovery. Besides, we know—from years of experience—that pursuing the causes of an eating disorder is a journey without end. There are usually multiple triggers and factors that contribute to an eating disorder, not one single cause, and it's a waste of much-needed time and energy to focus on the past.

That said, each scenario in this book does focus on a single particular trigger involved in the development of an eating disorder. However, we want to underscore that this was done only for the purposes of clarity, and that in real life, contributing factors are multiple, complicated, and immeasurable. Yes, we want to bring awareness to these triggers, so that eating disorders can be more easily averted. But please, waste no time on attempts to place blame or to trace the causality of the eating disorder affecting your life—that's history. However, understanding the purpose the eating disorder serves may enable parents and teens to discover healthier coping strategies. We entreat you to maintain a forward-looking focus, toward solutions and recovery.

HOW TO USE THIS BOOK

Conquering Eating Disorders is different from many other books on this subject for a couple of reasons. First of all, it is meant for both parents *and* teens—in fact, this book can be read together, as a family. It's also meant for siblings, other family members, therapists, teachers, coaches, best friends—anyone whose life is touched by an eating disorder or disordered eating. In addition to encouraging adults to be honest about the impact of an eating disorder, and helping them to discover their own blind spots, we have put some of the responsibility for change on teens, who need to be open and share the pain they are experiencing. In this way, adults and teens become equal partners in the solution and the recovery process.

But perhaps the major distinguishing element of this book is its unique format, which emphasizes the power of the story. We chose this format very intentionally. Stories reach people in an emotional way—often on an unconscious level—bypassing the intellectualizing we use to avoid painful feelings. We hope that by reading this collection of fictional first-person accounts, you will be able to empathize with the voices in this book, and the stories will resonate with your own experiences, touching your heart and mind.

Those suffering from an eating disorder, or disordered eating, may encounter a scenario with a story similar to their own, and see their hopes and fears echoed in those pages. Adults can read these stories and better understand what is going on in the minds and hearts of struggling teens. We hope that teens using this book eventually find the power and confidence to use their own voices, but in the meantime, this book, and the stories in it, can act as a bridge to cross the communication gap that almost always exists between adults and eating-disordered teens.

Though fictional, the voices are based on years of careful listening to our clients and their parents as they describe the private hell of fighting the fear of gaining weight, the gut-wrenching bingeing and purging, and the social isolation. Embedded in the stories are secret thoughts and strangled emotions seeking an outlet for expression.

Some of the teens in these stories are struggling with bulimia nervosa, characterized by eating binges followed by induced vomiting, laxative and diuretic abuse, fasting, and/or excessive exercise. Other stories are about teens exhibiting signs of anorexia nervosa, which involves unhealthy weight loss, distorted body image, cessation of menstrual periods, and, in some cases, bingeing and purging. Still other stories show teens suffering from compulsive overeating, which is eating without regard to hunger or fullness but in response to emotional need or stress. Binge-eating disorder is also addressed and is different from classic bulimia nervosa in that there is no compensatory behavior like vomiting, laxative abuse, or overexercising to counteract the binges. The binge-eating episodes are accompanied by extreme body dissatisfaction, shame, and sometimes obesity.

Some of the teens in our stories are girls, and some are boys. Some are athletes, and some are not. Some are from intact families, and others are from divorced families. Most important, each of these teens needs help, first from parents and caring adults, and in many cases, from professionals. Even when a professional is needed, the parental role—that of the supportive, empowering, unconditionally loving adult—is critical in the recovery process.

In each scenario you'll find a poignant story—usually from a teen, but sometimes from an adult—in which the eating disorder's major trigger becomes self-evident.

Following the story is a section called Points to Ponder, where you'll find a recounting of the elements of the scenario and an in-depth discussion of the trigger involved. Together, the scenario and Points to Ponder can help the reader to discover hidden motivations, as well as methods for unlocking feelings. In this section, we also offer suggestions about how the teens and the parents might have been helped, and we pose questions for the readers to deliberate, either individually or together.

In closing, each scenario features two sets of action points—one for parents, and one for teens—giving practical advice to apply to your own life situations. Here you'll find ways to shift attitudes and to have honest, courageous conversations that create possibilities for change and recovery.

In addition to the individual scenarios, the appendix has more information and tools to help bridge communication gaps and create an environment of healing and love.

WARNING SIGNS & SYMPTOMS

It may seem amazing that a parent can live with a teen and not know that he or she has been bingeing and purging for months— or even years. But this is not out of the ordinary. The onset of anorexia, for example, can be so gradual that the weight loss isn't noticed or acknowledged until it becomes drastic. To complicate matters, it is often difficult to distinguish an eating disorder from the normal hormonal and developmental ups and downs of adolescence. Sometimes a parent's own fear and close proximity to the problem may cause him or her to retreat into denial when initial symptoms appear, and as a result, coaches and teachers may notice these alarming symptoms before parents have become fully conscious of them. Teens are often ambivalent about being discovered. On the one hand, they are often very clever, working hard to conceal the indicators. But on the other hand, they are secretly hoping someone will notice, and they may feel dejected if no one does. For these reasons, it's very important for adults to arm themselves with as much information as possible about the potential triggers, warning signs, and symptoms associated with eating disorders.

Since parents live with their teens, they may sense that something just isn't right. To these parents: Trust your intuition. It is better to overreact than to miss an important cry for help. If you become alarmed, take your teen to the doctor or emergency room.

Many of the signs of an eating disorder are behavioral. Teens may show a decrease in desire for social interaction. For example, a daughter who has always been open and honest can suddenly become secretive or deceptive. She may disappear into the bathroom after eating, both at home and in restaurants. She might be irritable at mealtime, or may refuse to eat certain foods (usually high-fat foods). She may begin to stay home instead of going out with her friends. Visits to relatives may suddenly be met with resistance, although she has always loved these visits in the past. A teen may exercise excessively, preferring a workout to being with friends and family. Grades may suddenly drop, because the teen is having trouble concentrating or thinking clearly, due to low energy.

More serious signs are physiological: blue nail beds, dizziness, passing out, extreme fatigue, sleeplessness, and the absence of menstrual periods. If she is becoming bulimic, she may have swollen salivary glands that show up as "chipmunk cheeks." If she is becoming anorexic, she may begin losing hair on her head while developing fine hair on her body. This is a survival response, as her body is trying to conserve energy and keep her warm. She may begin to wear baggy clothes to hide her diminishing frame. She may also be experiencing (and concealing) chest pains caused by low potassium levels. You need to be most concerned about dehydration and electrolyte imbalance because both can put strain on the heart. Excessive exercise, coupled with little food and drink, can be especially dangerous because of the risk of dehydration and cardiac arrest.

Coaches may become concerned and notice a drive to excel that leads to decreased athletic performance and/or more frequent injuries. Weight loss may be encouraged by a coach to improve performance, but the teen can take it to dangerous extremes. Teammates may approach the coach after observing excessive weighing in the locker room or overhearing a purging episode that the eating-disordered friend is trying to hide. Teachers may detect the problem by noticing a sudden drop in grades, waning interest, or drowsiness in the classroom.

Adolescents can easily believe that danger lurks for others, but not for them. They often feel invincible, and teens with eating disorders ignore the realities in order to stay wedded to the perceived rescuer. Threats from parents or counselors about serious health problems or death are usually ineffective. As recovery progresses, they often give up this denial and may become truly frightened for a period of time. The reality that they *could* have died is terrifying, and feelings of being invincible turn to feelings of extreme vulnerability. Teenagers in the recovery process need to understand that these feelings are actually an indication of progress, and that they can be healed in time.

THE LIGHT AT THE END OF THE TUNNEL

We want to reassure you that people can recover from eating disorders, including those who have struggled for a prolonged period of time. When parents are supportive, and professional help is competent and caring, recovery is even more likely. When parents, teachers, coaches, and other adults can reach out to these young people in the early stages and reduce or prevent serious medical problems, relationship damage, and delayed development, prospects for recovery are all the greater. Best of all is when the eating-disordered teen gains the confidence and learns the tools to engage in conversations that will lead to wholeness and connection—tools that last a lifetime.

To truly make a difference, this process requires complete honesty and compelling courage. We understand your fears, and we know that it often seems easier to pretend the problem doesn't exist than to make the commitment to win this battle. But by working *together* on healing, parents and teens can empower each other, reduce heartbreak and build strong, deep relationships that will last a lifetime.

We celebrate your courage and offer to walk with you as you cross the bridge to recovery.

1. William D. McArdle, Frank I. Katch, and Victor Katch, *Sports and Exercise Nutrition* (Philadelphia: Lippincott, Williams and Wilkins, 2005), 512.

2. Abigail Natenshon, "Disordered Eating: Time for a Wake-Up Call," www.empoweredparents.com/1diagnosis/diagnosis_02.htm (accessed April 15, 2008).

FACTS AND STORY

Facts, facts everywhere
spoken, paper, digital, visual
racing past
swiftly crashing like waves of a restless sea.

Facts without connection
battering rams
breaking down the silence
of one's space.

Facts touched by story
connected and remade to form truth.

Story . . .
a thread that is sometimes golden
sometimes charred

yet weaving a path
through darkness into light.

Story . . .
precious story
holding us as people
holding us . . . connected
and open.

To hold one's story
with honor
with respect.

To know that one's story, and
its connection to the people
has roots
has connection
has redemption.

To be held in the stories of our people;
To know that Wakan-Taka* has walked with you,
To know that embrace of a higher power
Even as one feels the depth of loss.

To know the embrace of story . . .
like a blanket in cold winds,
knowing the gift of warmth and holding.

To be held in one's story
is to know
there is an end to isolation
to know that in the darkest part of the forest
we do not walk alone.

—*Jim Francek*
2001

*Wakan-Taka: "The Great Spirit" in the language of the Sioux nation
of North Dakota

Scenario 1

LOST IN THE FOG

WHEN A PARENT IS DEPRESSED

Light shines in darkness, because what else could it shine in?
— Alan Watts

Depression is a pandemic problem in our society, affecting millions of Americans each year. More than just "the blues," depression is very real and can be immobilizing when it reaches severe levels. Sufferers feel hopeless, helpless, and sometimes suicidal, and are often unable to cope with parenting and other daily pressures.

When parents become depressed, there is a serious trickle-down effect on their children. Depressed adults crave isolation and are easily overwhelmed, so it's easy to see why depressed parents might not want to deal with their children's personal problems when they themselves feel barely able to keep their own heads above water. This leaves the teens of depressed parents to cope for themselves at a time when they need reassurance and advice the most. Oftentimes, because of the stigma attached to depression, parents resist getting professional help, and as a result, their children can become depressed and question whether there is any relief in sight. This is a point at which teens might seek alternative ways to numb their feelings of despair or to make up for a lack of nurturing.

In the following scenario, fourteen-year-old Debbie struggles with her mother's "headaches," which are actually a front for depression. She hopes for her mother's attention and, when it is not forthcoming, figures out her own way of soothing herself.

IN SOME WAYS, THE WALK HOME TODAY was the same as it is every day—ten minutes, two blocks, borrrrring. But today, it wasn't just boring. It was awful. My geometry and chemistry books were as heavy as my heart. How could David just tell me it was over? Just like that, with no explanation? I didn't understand any of it. I wondered whether there was something horribly wrong with me. Something so horrible that no one wanted to tell me—but instead just broke up with me.

No matter how much I hoped it would be different, coming home was the same that day as it was every day. The kitchen light was out, *as usual.* The house was dark and uninviting, *as usual.* No one came to the door to greet me, *as usual.* I couldn't seem to catch a break! It was the worst day of my entire life, and by all indications, Mom was hiding away in her dark bedroom with one of her "headaches," *as usual.*

I wondered what would happen if I told Mom how much I missed how she used to be waiting for me to come home from school. How she'd pour me a glass of juice and we'd munch on pretzels while I told her about my day. How we used to have dinner together. How much I miss making her laugh. How much I miss *her.* She'd probably think I was being lame. I'm too old to have those kinds of feelings anyway. Aren't I?

What if I told Mom I know her headaches aren't real— that I know she is just depressed? Who is she trying to kid, anyway? I wish she would just admit it—at least then we could talk about it. She must think I'm a baby, too young to understand. Or too stupid.

I could've just gone to my room and started my homework, but I knew there was no way I could concentrate. I was a complete mess, and my mind was racing. *How am I going to deal?* I kept thinking. *How am I going to go to school every day, and have to face him? I feel like my life is over, and I'm only fourteen!*

I didn't know what to do. I had to talk to someone, anyone! But I was too embarrassed to call a friend. I didn't want it to get around school how upset I was—how much I was crying because of David.

I put my books down and tiptoed up the stairs toward the bedroom. *Maybe,* I thought, *Mom won't have one of her so-called headaches today. Or even if she does, maybe she'll see how much I've been crying and ask me what's wrong. Maybe she'll finally rally. Maybe today would be one of her better days,* I thought. *Maybe she'd at least be awake and reading.*

No such luck. When I got to her door, I saw that her light was off. But by then, I was desperate. I didn't care whether she was sleeping. If I didn't get this off my chest, I felt like I would die. I quietly opened the door and stood in the doorway. But before I even got one word out, she waved me away, saying, "Debbie, honey, let me sleep. I feel awful. My head is killing me. Go get something to eat, and get your homework started."

I turned and headed straight for the kitchen. I didn't even bother to turn on the light. *Let the house be dark,* I thought. *Just like Mom. Just like me.* I grabbed the package of Oreos and stuffed three cookies in my mouth at once. Then I went for more. At first they tasted good, but then I didn't even taste them. I didn't care about what they tasted like. I just stuffed them in my mouth. Once I'd devoured the whole package, I went for a bag of chips. Next came two bowls of frosted cereal.

The whole time I was eating, I felt nothing anymore. I was good and numb. As soon as it was over, though, the panic started to set in. But I knew how to get rid of that feeling too. I headed straight for the bathroom. After I got rid of all that damage, I had that pure, empty feeling. I actually felt *good.* I felt light. I went to my bedroom to look at myself in the mirror, to make sure I wasn't fat. I checked my hipbones to make sure they were still sticking out. Then I pulled the scale out from underneath my bed, took a deep breath, and stepped up onto it. I let out a big sigh. I was okay.

I was actually *glad* now that I didn't have to get Mom involved. Why would I want to add to her sorrows? And as far as I was concerned, David could take a hike. I went downstairs again and grabbed my textbooks. I turned on the light in the dining room and started my homework. I felt exhausted in a way, but I also had a sense that everything was going to be okay.

POINTS TO PONDER

Debbie was feeling alone and was looking for comfort because she faced a personal rejection. But because of the feelings of isolation and alienation that accompany depression, Debbie's mother was either unable to detect how much her daughter needed her attention—or possibly, due to the sometimes all-consuming nature of depression, her mother's natural ability to empathize was compromised.

In the absence of a listening ear, food became a soothing but fleeting substitute for the attention Debbie needed. The taste of food is immediately gratifying, and when overeating reaches the level of bingeing, the process can become mindless and numbing. Painful feelings temporarily disappear, and problems shrink in importance. However, there is the inevitable desire to purge the food after a binge, when the fear of weight gain sets in. Vomiting or laxative abuse can seem to be the perfect answer, but they only perpetuate the problem and can lead to a cycle of bingeing and purging that becomes an entrenched eating disorder.

So what went wrong here? Unfortunately, as it often does, the power of depression created a vast divide between two people—a mother and her daughter. Had either the mother or the daughter reached out to bridge this communication gap, this scenario might have had a much more constructive ending. Even though Debbie's mother was depressed, it would have made a tremendous difference if she had called Debbie into her room to talk to her, to see her face—even for a few minutes. In that time, Debbie's mother might have realized—despite her own depression—that her daughter desperately needed her. Once that realization was made, Debbie's mother could have told her that she needed a little bit of time to collect herself—to take a shower perhaps, or to wash her face, or to have Debbie bring her some soothing tea—so that they could talk.

By the same token, it might have made a tremendous difference had Debbie persisted with her mother, saying, "I know you're feeling awful, but I am too, and I really need to be comforted and to talk to you about it. What can I do to help you feel well enough to listen?" In this scenario, it seems quite clear that Debbie's mother had no idea that her daughter was in such an emotional state when she came to the bedroom. Had her mother known, she may have been able to put her depression aside and come to the aid of her daughter, who was in need.

When thinking about what could have been done differently in this scenario, the first thing that needs to be addressed is the fact that Debbie's mother was apparently not getting help for her depression. She may not have known that depression is very treatable, both with therapy and with antidepressant medication. It was vital for her to seek professional help, not only for the benefit of her own mental health, but also for the health of Debbie, who was feeling the effects of her mother's depression and suffering with her.

If depressed parents don't receive help, teens can develop numerous problems and compulsive behaviors, only one of them being an eating disorder. Because professional help is readily available, and because most people respond to treatment rather quickly, there is no reason to suffer so chronically. As difficult as it might at first seem, depressed parents will benefit tremendously by putting aside any shame or stigma attached to being depressed, taking medications, or seeing a therapist. Even doing so for a set term of a few months can clear the fog enough to reveal a light at the end of the tunnel.

The second thing that needs to be addressed is that it is almost always healthier for a parent to tell a teenager that he or she is depressed, rather than to hide it. Teens are highly intuitive, and if they sense a parent is reluctant to talk about something, they will assume that it's too terrible to bring up. Often they suspect that it's even worse than it actually is. Many teens—especially those prone to eating disorders—are very empathetic and are afraid to bring up subjects they feel might be hurtful to their parents. Parents may do well to share with their teenagers the fact that they want to get help for their depression, and that they would like their understanding. But it should be made very clear to the teen that the parent is not going to be relying on the teen to feel better. An open conversation about the depression, and about the plan of action being taken, will allow both parent and teen some freedom and agency to take care of themselves.

Parents may assume that their teens know their love is unconditional, but children need tangible expressions of this love—particularly during the teen years, when so many challenges and hormonal changes are occurring. Some teenagers are barely affected by the moods and problems of their parents; others are highly sensitive and easily affected by them. Sensitive teens can feel guilty and responsible for fixing the problem if parents do not seek help. They can turn to an eating disorder to control what they feel they *can* control, or to numb the pain.

In comparison to the kinds of challenges and problems that most adults face, a teenager's problems might seem negligible. But parents must keep in mind that these problems do not *feel* negligible to the teen; in fact, they often seem overwhelming and, if unresolved, become formidable barriers to developing a healthy identity and self-confidence.

When they were teens themselves, some parents may have been fortunate enough to have come home from school and found refuge after receiving an F on a test, having a fight with a boyfriend, hearing critical words from a well-intentioned teacher, or not making the cheerleading squad. Home may have been a place to unburden themselves from the frustrations of the day, to feel unconditionally loved, and to renew their sagging self-esteem by being comforted and encouraged.

Some adults, however, did not find a refuge at home and lacked a role model who could teach them to listen without judgment and put aside distractions and personal problems to help another person in need. It is harder for such adults to realize the power they have to help their children. And if depression enters the picture, these adults can find it even harder to reach out to their teens—to communicate and break the cycle of silence.

The good news is, it *is possible* for parents to learn how to get in sync with their teens, even if their depression and lack of good role models are part of the equation. When a teen comes home from school, it is important for a parent to notice her face and the mood it shows. Taking a few minutes to listen to her and comfort her if she needs to be comforted can bolster her self-esteem and help her to feel connected and loved. Preparing a healthy snack for her on a regular basis puts food in the right perspective and teaches her to use food as nourishment, not as a substitute for love. Sometimes just a few minutes of focusing on her and her only is all she needs, and she can begin her homework, having experienced her parent's availability and love.

Part of the solution can be talking honestly about the depression and not hiding behind a headache or another excuse.

Explaining the problem truthfully and declaring the intention to get help can be the reassurance that a teen needs to have hope that things will get better.

Teens can also take some initiative in this situation and can call ahead by cell phone to let parents know they need some time to talk. They can ask a depressed parent with a headache what they can do to help and can get some aspirin or offer encouraging words when they arrive at home.

With very intentional actions on the part of a parent—despite the depression—and an attempt by the teen to reach out to a parent, the improved and open communication can become a healing bond between them. The need for disordered eating is reduced or eliminated and is replaced by the more powerful force of love and understanding. This process can take time to feel natural. It takes persistent effort to break the silence and to build the trust that fortifies teens against the need for an eating disorder to speak for them.

CHANGING THE PATTERN

PARENTS

✒ If you suspect you are depressed, get help. Contact a doctor or a therapist as soon as possible. You *deserve* to feel better, and your health and the health of your children depend on it.

❧ Tell your children that you are suffering from depression, but that it's okay and that you are getting help. Also let them know that you may need some extra help and understanding from them while you are in the process of recovering.

❧ Make sure your children know that it is not their responsibility to cure you of depression; that you are taking care of it yourself.

❧ Make sure your children know that it is not their fault that you are depressed.

❧ Tell your children in no uncertain terms that they are important enough for you to drop what you are doing and listen if they are having an emotional emergency. Let them know that it is okay to persist in asking for what they need if they are not getting it from you.

❧ When you are troubled, practice coming back to the *present moment* and focusing on one person or task at a time.

❧ Be patient with yourself; recovery from depression may at times seem slow.

⮞   Make it a point to check in with your children each day, face to face. You may even find that actively listening to your loved ones takes your mind off your own thoughts.

⮞   Remember to say "I love you." Depression often makes us forget to say such things, but your children need to hear it, especially during this time.

TEENS

⮞   If your parent is depressed, try to understand that they may not be as responsive to your needs as you feel they should be. Try to be patient, but know that you can gently persist when you are not getting what you need.

⮞   Know that it is *not* your fault that your parent is depressed.

⮞   Know that it is *not* your responsibility to cure your parent of depression.

⮞   Give your parents a chance to hear your feelings. Tell them what is bothering you, and trust that they care very much, even if it may not seem like it right away.

⮞   If your parents seem preoccupied, tell them that you want their undivided attention for a few minutes. You deserve to be heard.

∾   Do your part to communicate as clearly as possible about what you need.

∾   Remember to say "I love you." It helps tremendously.

SUPPLEMENTARY READING

FOR PARENTS

Feeling Good, by David Burns

Mind over Mood: Change How You Feel by Changing the Way You Think, by Dennis Greenberger and Christine Padesky

Reinventing Your Life, by Jeffrey E. Young

Thoughts and Feelings: Taking Control of Your Moods and Your Life, by Matthew McKay, Martha Davis, and Patrick Fanning

Parenting Well When You're Depressed: A Complete Resource for Maintaining a Healthy Family, by Alexis D. Henry, Jonathan C. Clayfield, Susan M. Phillips, and Joanne Nicholson

Scenario 2

GREAT EXPECTATIONS

WHEN TEENS ARE PRESSURED TO MEND A PARENT'S BROKEN DREAMS

If you can lessen your expectation (even a little bit) about how things are supposed to be, and instead open your heart and acceptance to what is, you'll be well on your way to a calmer and much happier life.

—Richard Carlson, PhD

Many parents have well-intentioned goals to give their teens a life that they never had. Sometimes, however, those intentions can take the form of pressure to engage in activities that their children don't actually enjoy. In such cases, the teens are in a double bind, conflicted between pleasing their parents and pleasing themselves.

All teens at some level want to make their parents proud of them. Afraid of disappointing them—or even afraid of losing their love—they may feel anxious about taking a stand against an activity or sport their parents decided they should love. If family communication is not open, it is even harder to object to the activity.

In this scenario, fifteen-year-old Tracey is caught in this exact bind. Out of a sense of obligation to her father, she spends most of her free time playing a sport she is good at but doesn't enjoy.

EVER SINCE I COULD REMEMBER, BASKETBALL

had been my life. But there was one problem: I hated, hated, *hated* basketball! I hated talking about it, I hated going to the games, and I hated practicing layups and running drills every single day. All I wanted to do after school was go home and relax and watch *Oprah* like a normal person. And besides, what teenage girl in her right mind wants to be known as the chick who plays on three basketball leagues?

But no one even noticed that I wasn't into it. My father and my brother, Scott, worshipped basketball so much that they were completely blind to how much I couldn't stand it. It was as if they couldn't even conceive of the fact that their very own flesh-and-blood relative did not eat, drink, sleep, and live the sport. They didn't even notice that my enthusiasm was totally nonexistent, and that made *me* feel nonexistent.

I guess I could have said something, but I didn't have the heart—or the courage—to tell Dad I wanted to quit. I'd been playing the game since the third grade, when he first taught me to dribble. Since then, he'd come to every single game Scott and I ever played. He cheered us on from the sidelines and videotaped every one of our plays so that he could later point out ways to improve.

The end result? Both Scott and I got to be really good. Great, even. I didn't think Dad would ever be able to understand how someone so good at basketball could have dreams of quitting. His own dream when he was younger was to be a basketball star. But that didn't happen, and he never explained why. It was always mysterious to me, and one thing was clear: If he didn't tell us about it, it meant he didn't want to talk about it. Maybe he was ashamed of it. Whatever the reason, I knew better than to ask. The last thing in the world I ever wanted was to make him sad or disappointed in me. Some of my happiest moments were when I saw my dad's eyes light up after I made a foul shot.

But my daily practice was making me look like Scott! I didn't *want* big strong thighs and bulging calf muscles! I wanted to have a body like the models in *Seventeen:* skinny legs, pale skin, and long slender necks. What a cool look! Every girl in school would die for a body like that. Plus, there's this boy, Justin, in my art class. I really like him. He is *really* cute. But why would he like me if I'm built like a boy?!

I knew I could get the perfect body if I tried hard enough. Dad taught me long ago that visualization is the key to achieving your goals. He proved to me how the act of imagining myself making the perfect shot is just as effective as hours of practice—if not even *more* effective. So why wouldn't it work just as well with getting skinny? I began to visualize myself being as thin as possible.

It was easy. Before long, hamburgers began to disgust me, and chips and pizza were so easy to resist that the pounds began to melt off. Then I started feeling shaky and weak at basketball practice, and my legs felt like jelly when I ran. But I liked the weak sensation. It was proof that I was getting skinny.

I guess things finally changed the day I blacked out at practice and hit the floor. When I came to, I didn't even remember how I got there. I was suddenly looking up at Dad's face. Normally so proud when he looked at me, his face was now gray and scared. He picked me up, carried me to the car, and headed for the emergency room. I didn't want to go, but I knew I needed help. I was dizzy and couldn't concentrate on what Dad was saying to me. I did hear him call my mother on the way and tell her to meet us at the hospital.

When we arrived at the hospital, the doctor started me on an IV and drew my blood. After a long wait for the results, she told us that my potassium was dangerously low, and that I was seriously dehydrated. She explained how hard this combination is on the heart, and that I was fortunate to have gotten to the hospital quickly. After asking me a few embarrassing questions about my eating, she told my parents that I was in the grips of a serious eating disorder and needed treatment. She sent us home with some therapists' names and told my parents that they needed to make sure I was eating and drinking. Basketball was out, she said, because strenuous exercise makes dehydration worse if a person is not eating very much. I was very relieved about not having to play basketball, but I didn't like the disappointed look on my father's face. He didn't argue, though, because I could tell that the doctor had scared him. My mother didn't say much. She just held my hand and told me everything would be all right.

Since I didn't have to play after that day, I came home after school and hung out in my room, watching TV and talking to Lexie, my poodle. Scott had gone back to college after semester break, so I didn't have him to talk to. My so-called friends only wanted to bug me about being too thin, and I didn't want to hear it. I knew they were just jealous. Now that Scott had left for college, I didn't feel close to anyone. And when Mom and Dad were home, they had long conversations in the family room. I didn't know whether they were talking about me, or Scott's grades, or whether they were just trying to figure out how to pay the bills. They seemed too wrapped up in each other to notice anything going on with me. All they did was force me to eat in front of them, like the doctor told them to do, which was fine. No problem! They had no idea I was throwing up everything I could when they weren't paying attention.

I was amazed. Grungy, sweaty basketball was over. Finally I felt free and in control of my life. Without even realizing it, I killed two birds with one stone. I got out of basketball, and

I got the body I wanted. Or almost. I still need to lose some more bulk.

And I never had to tell Dad how much I hate the sport he loves so much. These days he is either grim-faced or expressionless. I think he and Mom might be worried about my weight, but they never say anything about it. Sometimes I think I should tell them the truth—that I'm lonely, and that I'm making myself throw up—but I'm way too scared of how it would affect them.

POINTS TO PONDER

Like many girls who develop eating disorders, Tracey found it very difficult to communicate directly about her needs and her feelings. Instead, she communicated indirectly—and dangerously—by bringing on a physical crisis. Many girls who develop eating disorders are very intuitive and empathetic; again, Tracey fits this description.

Her intuition about her father's feelings may have been on target. It may have been true that he would have been extremely disappointed if she quit, and it may have been true that he was living vicariously through the basketball success of his children. But despite her intuition and empathy, what Tracey failed to see was how much *more* pain was caused by her eating disorder than ever would have been caused if she had just told her father the truth.

But Tracey's reluctance to communicate directly also appears to be a family-wide problem. Her father, though devoted, must not have been communicating very well either; otherwise, he would probably have noticed Tracey's waning enthusiasm for the sport. Also, the fact that he refrained from talking about what happened with his own basketball career testifies to a certain element of avoidance in the family. Tracey probably figured, from her parents' behavior, that it was not acceptable to talk about uncomfortable subject matters. So when she sensed—rightly or wrongly—that her dad *needed* her to play basketball to meet his unfulfilled dreams, she did not believe it was okay to check out this impression with her dad. We also see that although she has felt ignored and lonely since her brother left for college, she does not feel comfortable telling her parents about it. She seems to be protecting her parents from her dissatisfaction and protecting herself from their disappointment. She turns to her dog for comfort and retreats into an eating disorder.

But perhaps the most significant issue in this scenario was the fact that Tracey's father was not able to see his goals as separate from Tracey's. With all good intentions, he mistook his needs for hers. Had he attempted to be more in touch with Tracey's true desires and needs, he would have been more apt to pick up on the signs that basketball was no longer fun for her.

Perhaps he *did* sense that Tracey did not want to play any longer but underestimated the importance of the situation. Perhaps he figured Tracey's declining interest was just a phase, brought on by puberty and peer pressures. And perhaps that was a correct assessment. However, the critical factor—open, honest communication—was not present, and that's why an uncomfortable matter turned into a life-threatening one.

An eating disorder can easily become a way to say what a person cannot say or is afraid to say directly. In this case, Tracey knows what she is having trouble saying: *I don't want to play basketball. I want time for other things.* Her eating disorder speaks for her and gives her parents a reason to tell her she must quit basketball. It was a desperate ploy to be loyal to her father at the expense of her own welfare.

Open and honest family communication can offer a dose of extra protection against the onset of an eating disorder. Mothers and fathers who dedicate themselves to this kind of honesty are giving their teens a priceless gift. By the same token, teens who risk assertiveness and say what they need are helping their parents to understand them better.

CHANGING THE PATTERN

PARENTS

❧   Check in with yourself, honestly. Do you have hopes that your child will fulfill a dream that you once had for yourself? If so, admit that to yourself and decide that you will not expect your child to follow your dreams.

❧   Pay attention to the ways your teen is becoming a truly unique person, different from you and anyone else.

❧ Suggest that you and your teen each write down all of your interests and goals for the future, and then talk about the ways you are different from each other.

❧ There are other ways to heal broken dreams. If you were never able to excel in a sport, or to be an actor, join a local sports league or try out for a part in a local play. Your dreams are still important, and engaging in your own interests will help avoid living vicariously through your children.

TEENS

❧ Remember: You have a right to have your own interests and your own personality.

❧ Never make assumptions about how your parents will react before you have talked to them. You may be wrong about what they are thinking.

❧ As hard as it seems, work up the courage to talk to your parents when you don't want to pursue an interest of theirs. They would rather know the truth than have you risk your safety because you are holding back your feelings.

❧ When you talk to them, use the words, "I feel" or "I want" so that you are speaking for yourself and not blaming them.

Even if the first few conversations don't go perfectly, you have given your family a gift by opening up honest communication.

Scenario 3

"WHO AM I *NOW?*"

WHEN A TEEN FACES A
SUDDEN IDENTITY CRISIS

The journey in between what you once were and who you are
now becoming is where the dance of life really takes place.
—Barbara De Angelis

The teen years are a crucial time to begin to establish a sense of identity. Teens usually experiment with lots of different activities in the process of choosing what they are good at and most enjoy. However, they sometimes become overly dependent on one activity to define themselves. When an unexpected event such as an injury makes pursuit of that interest impossible, some teens are prone to choosing an unhealthy outlet for their unmet needs, especially when family communication is not open.

If competition is part of the picture, teens can find themselves in the grips of an eating disorder, which is attractive because of the competitive pursuit of thinness and body perfection. The eating disorder is unhealthy, both physically and emotionally, and represents a desperate attempt to regain a sense of self. Unfortunately, it also closes off other avenues that could provide new and healthier ways to forge an even stronger sense of identity.

In the following scenario, sixteen-year-old John has just found out that he is no longer able to play hockey. As a result, he begins the relentless pursuit of thinness to substitute for the self-esteem he derived from his success at hockey.

––––––––––––––––––––

MY ENTIRE BODY WENT NUMB, AND THE

doctor's words were ringing in my ears. I knew I was in shock. All of a sudden, my hockey career was officially over, and there was nothing I could do or say about it.

I'd been warned months ago that one more knee injury would mean the end of hockey for me, so I was more careful than ever. But in hockey, there's only so much you can do to protect yourself from getting hurt. Then, two weeks ago, at the state championships, a guy from the other team sidelined me when I was about to make a goal. I hit the ice—hard—and my knee hurt pretty bad. Whatever, I was used to that. But when Mom saw me still limping a week later, she took me to the doctor, even though I told her it was fine. After some tests, the doctor said that not only had I torn another ligament in my knee, but that because of a congenital abnormality, I was particularly prone to knee injuries. And then he handed me my fate: I was no longer to play hockey, or any other contact sport, for the rest of my life.

I felt a black fog descend over me and left the doctor's office alternating between shock and devastation. As Mom and I walked toward the car, my legs felt like jelly. I focused on putting one foot in front of the other, hoping I would make it without collapsing. My whole world seemed rocked to the core. *How could I possibly go on?* I thought.

Almost the whole way home, Mom didn't say a word. She's always silent when her feelings are intense. I could sense her distress, but I was afraid that if I said anything, I would upset her more. Maybe she was worried about the same thing—afraid talking would upset *me* more. And I had a sinking feeling of dread at the thought of having to tell Dad the news when he got home from work later that day. He had been so proud of me. I knew he would never think less of me, and I knew he would try to downplay it all and focus on the positive, but deep inside, he would be disappointed beyond belief.

So much was going through my mind during that car ride home. The future was never scary to me before. It was never an unknown. Now, all of a sudden, it was a mystery to me. Before this, everyone always knew I was scholarship material, and that hockey was my ticket to college. But now, here I was, about to become a senior in high school, and I no longer had any *clue* about who I was or what I was going to do with my life! *What do I even have to look forward to?* I thought.

I decided, right there in the car, not to tell the team about this until there was no other choice. As far as the guys knew, I was just recuperating from an injury, and I was going to let them keep thinking that. I thanked God it was summer and I didn't have to go to practice for a long time. The thought of any of those guys feeling sorry for me was way more than I could handle. I realized I didn't even want to hang out with them. I didn't even want to see their faces. *So what am I going to do with myself all summer?* I wondered.

Suddenly Mom's voice broke into my thoughts and said, "John, do you want to stop and get a chocolate milkshake on the way home?" I knew it was her way of saying she felt sad for me. Milkshakes were my favorite, and she knew it. But the thought of it made me sick. In fact, food seemed disgusting. Suddenly I was struck by a bolt of fear that took my breath away: *Without sports, would I become fat and ugly?* I had a huge appetite and was as famous for the pizza I could put away after a game as I was for my speed on the ice. My friends were always saying I was as thin as a rail, but what if they had just been saying that? For the first time, I began to realize that I need to watch what I eat. I decided that I would spend the next couple of months making sure I didn't get fat. *Maybe I should even lose some weight,* I thought.

Once the boredom of summer set in, I thought I would go crazy. But then I had my knee surgery, and *boom!* I lost weight easily. After that, I decided to challenge myself to see how little I could eat and how many pounds I could drop. I prided myself on keeping my stomach flat and my ribs protruding. I checked both areas when I got up in the morning and before I went to bed. Within a month, I lost twenty pounds. I congratulated myself on being as good at this weight-loss thing as I had been at hockey. Competition is just part of who I am, and I am on a roll.

The feelings of hopelessness and disappointment melt away more and more with each pound. I feel like I could do anything! And my parents don't even seem to notice anything different. But who can ever tell what they're thinking?

POINTS TO PONDER

The main factor in this scenario is John's perceived loss of identity. This loss—combined with his perceived lack of control over his fate, his naturally competitive nature, and his family's inability to communicate about difficult emotions—all contributed to John's slide toward anorexia.

John's entire identity had been his talent at hockey—this in and of itself was not particularly healthy. Even if John were able to continue playing, in the long term it would have been better for his sense of self to be more multifaceted and well rounded. But because the critical element of hockey was suddenly taken away from him, John experienced this event as the end of his identity as he knew it. Because he had not developed other interests or passions to bolster his self-esteem, he was devastated by the loss of hockey and the acclaim it had brought him.

This loss was accompanied by a perceived lack of control. John's perception was that his body and genetics had let him down by making him unusually susceptible to knee injury. He felt he had no control over his body and no control over the doctor's decision that he must stop playing contact sports. Anorexia or bulimia often emerges when a person feels out of control of his emotions and of his life. New ways of feeling in control need to be invented, and unfortunately, this sense of control can sometimes be achieved by focusing obsessively on food and calorie intake or by forcing oneself to lose weight.

John's naturally competitive nature no longer had an outlet, and since his summer appeared to be devoid of any new challenges, he devised his own way to compete, this time by losing weight. His family could have encouraged him to channel his competitive nature into directions that were safe for his knee. He could have started swimming competitively, run for school government, entered a fundraising walkathon, or found a creative outlet that enabled him to enter his work in contests. With his parents' encouragement, he could have discovered new aspects of his personality and begun to forge a new identity around interests and talents that he didn't know he possessed.

In addition to these challenges, the family dynamics were such that no one seemed to be accustomed to putting feelings into words and communicating in an emotionally intimate way. His mother's offer to stop for a milkshake showed that she sincerely wanted to find a way to soothe John, but her silence about what was actually going on created an atmosphere of anxiety: John had to guess at what she was feeling, figure out if it was okay to express his emotions, and wonder what he could do for *her.* In addition, John felt that his father swas not going to be forthcoming about his thoughts and feelings about the bad news either. This lack of honest communication carries implicit, underlying messages: "This is too hard to talk about. I'm afraid to talk about it with you. This situation is a taboo subject."

Participation in sports releases endorphins that can help with emotional pain and take up some of the slack when feelings have no natural outlet. In John's case, his family's pattern of communicating indirectly and withholding feelings may have set the stage for his increased dependence on sports, which served as an emotional outlet. When this outlet became blocked, he was left without an adequate coping mechanism.

The tremendous loss John felt at losing his identity as a hockey player might have been lessened were he able to talk about his greatest fears: "Who am I now? Am I going to be fat? How am I going to get into college? What do I have to look forward to?" It is likely that if John's parents had opened up, he might have followed suit. He might have voiced these scary questions out loud, and found out that their answers were not as terrifying as they seemed in the silence of his own mind. His parents could have helped him recognize that his identity was *not* based on hockey only; that he had many other talents and assets. They could have reassured him that he was not at all overweight, and had no need for concern about becoming fat, and they could have encouraged him to take up a low-impact, non-contact sport such as swimming to fuel his competitive drive and alleviate his fears about gaining weight. They could have explained that a hockey scholarship was not the only way for him to go to college and reminded him of all the countless experiences he had to look forward to.

When teens need to make drastic adaptations as a result of injury or other unexpected events that rock their sense of who they are, a little bit of encouragement from parents to talk about vulnerable emotions can go a long way. A courageous step from John to open the communication may have been all his parents needed to begin listening to his struggle.

It doesn't matter who begins the honest conversation, it just matters that *someone* opens the door to what can be a fruitful discussion. Such a discussion can help teens going through an identity crisis, to channel their needs in a positive direction and regain their sense of self.

CHANGING THE PATTERN

PARENTS

∾   If your teen has suffered an identity crisis, encourage him to talk about it and share any fears he might have.

❧ Make sure to share your own feelings about your teen's loss, remembering that silence breeds anxiety. It is better for him to know how you feel than for him to fear the worst. You provide a healthy example and build trust by sharing your own vulnerable thoughts and feelings.

❧ Listen to your teen's feelings without trying to change them. Let him know that it is normal to feel sad after a personal loss, and that it is healthy to express those emotions. This point is *particularly* important for male teens, who often get messages from society that it is unmanly to express sadness.

❧ If your teen seems to be particularly focused on one aspect of his identity, remind him of all the other things that make him an interesting and exciting person. Encourage him to be well-rounded in his interests.

❧ Make sure your teen knows that it is not his responsibility to take care of your feelings, even when those feelings have to do with his own life and future.

❧ Do everything you can to create an atmosphere of open communication in your family, and make sure nothing is "too taboo" to talk about. Open communication and mutual expression of feelings are the most vital keys to derailing an eating disorder.

TEENS

❦ Instead of focusing on an unexpected and unwelcome change as a bad thing, try to see it as an opportunity to reinvent yourself. Now is the time to daydream about what the next chapter of your life is going to be like.

❦ Who you are is so much more than "one thing." Take some time to read about famous athletes, scholars, politicians, and celebrities. You'll quickly find that those who are happiest and most successful are the ones who have many different interests.

❦ Ask your friends and family members what they think your strengths and interests are. You may be surprised to learn that you loved drawing in elementary school or showed an interest in science or math that you never had time to pursue.

❦ Make a decision to try a new activity that you have never explored, such as fishing or cooking. Read all you can about it, and dare to experiment with the first steps to achieving some success.

❦ Always talk to your family and friends about your feelings when you are devastated by a turn of events, even if it feels scary in the beginning. It will become easier, and you will become closer to everyone in the process. Give your friends and family the gift of being able to help you by showing how much they care.

Scenario 4

THE FAMILY'S GOOD NAME

WHEN TEENS ARE EXPECTED TO
KEEP UP APPEARANCES

People are like stained-glass windows. They sparkle when the sun is out, but when the darkness sets in, their true beauty is revealed only if there is light from within.

—Dr. Elisabeth Kübler-Ross

There is a tremendous amount of pressure in our society today to keep up appearances. Neither parents nor teenagers are immune. Parents may feel the need to send their child to prestigious universities or colleges because that is what their friends and neighbors are doing. They may also feel their children need to dress a certain way, drive a certain kind of car, go to all the parties—or somehow, they have failed as parents. Teenagers usually feel pressure to look like their peers too—to wear name-brand clothing and be a part of the popular group at school. Often their biggest fear is being different or unique from their friends.

In this scenario, eighteen-year-old Sally is not the typical teen. She feels very different from her peers and is okay with that. She wants to go against the norm but runs into strong opposition from her parents.

IT WAS THE LAST DAY OF MY SUMMER JOB,

and it felt like the best part of my life was coming to a close. On a normal day, I loved my bike ride to the child care center where I worked—especially the part where I got to ride through the peaceful grounds of the botanical gardens, taking in the rainbow of beautiful flowers that cheered me on from the sides of the bike path.

But today my thoughts were elsewhere. Being with the children at the center always felt more like play than work, and I was going to miss their smiling little faces and squeals of laughter. All the people at the center were wonderful! But best of all was the director, Ms. Emma. She took me under her wing and taught me so much. She showed me how to reach out to the children who were shy or unwilling to participate in the day's activities. And when I got the idea to have the children bring in their favorite storybooks from home to share with the other children, Ms. Emma said, "That's a brilliant idea!" It made me feel so good that she admired the way I worked. For the first time in my life, I felt accepted and appreciated for who I am. For the first time, I felt like someone actually listened to my thoughts and opinions. For the first time, I felt like I could really make a difference in the world.

Ms. Emma was great. She was so understanding and such a good listener that for a while, I considered telling her about my secret. But then I realized it might change her opinion of me, that I might be a disappointment to her—a thought I couldn't bear. The whole thing was a mess, and not even Ms. Emma would be able to understand how desperate and disgusting I felt.

Only when I got off my bike did I realize I'd been crying the whole ride there. I quickly brushed the tears away, locked up my bike, and forced a smile as I entered the center. It's a good thing I did, because as soon as I walked in, I saw that everyone was there waiting for me with huge smiles on their faces. "Surprise!" they yelled out. The children couldn't contain their excitement and ran up to me screaming.

"They couldn't wait to see the look on your face," said Ms. Emma. "And they each drew a picture, just for you."

I was blown away. It was all I could do not to burst into tears again. I hugged each of the kids as they proudly handed me their pictures. "Wow, you guys, I can't believe you did all this for me!" I said. "Your pictures are beautiful! What a great surprise! Thank you so much."

I never would have thought a summer job could mean so much to me. I knew in my heart that my decision to work this summer was the best thing I ever could have done. My job at the child care center proved to me that what I suspected for so long is true: There *is* more to life than what people look like and how much money people make. But when I told Mom last spring I was going to get a summer job, she wasn't particularly thrilled, to say the least. "What about your tennis lessons, and all the parties before you go away to college?" she asked. I couldn't believe how clueless my mom was!

"Mom, have you forgotten how miserable I was after every party I went to last summer?" I asked. "I hated those parties. And you know I don't particularly like playing tennis. I'm not really good at it either."

Fortunately, for once, Dad sided with me: "It'll be good for her to work and earn a little pocket money," he said. "It'll teach her the value of time and money." In the end, I was "allowed" to work. I was so relieved! By that point, just the thought of wasting another summer—playing tennis and lying around the pool, listening to Sherry and Kate gossip and obsess about their bodies and worry about what to wear to the next party—made me sick.

I worked hard all summer, and I loved it. My job gave me a sense of responsibility I'd never felt before, and I felt proud to be so independent. By the end of the summer, I'd saved more than $3,000. It felt great to know that I had some money of my own, and that I could save it or use it on whatever

I wanted. I'd been thinking about doing a semester abroad once I started college—maybe even Australia, where my dad is from—and I knew that my money would help me with all the additional expenses that would come with living and traveling in another country.

Last spring, even though I said I didn't want to, Mom and Dad insisted that we all pile in the car and drive up and down the East Coast to look at some of the top colleges. I wanted to go to a state university, but Mom was determined for me to go to one of those schools where girls from "good" families go. "After all," she said, "what would people think if you just went to a state university? They would probably think we can't afford a private college!"

While we were on our whirlwind tour, I stayed in the dorm at St. Joseph College, the one my Mom had fallen in love with. It was awful. All the girls asked me about was what sorority I was going to pledge and what my daddy did for a living. They never even asked me anything *real*—like what I liked to do or what I was going to major in. It felt just like what I had endured my whole life: trying to live up to some sort of artificial image. But it didn't seem to matter what I thought, or how terrible my experience at St. Joseph had been. It was pretty clear: I was going to have little if any say in my own future. Before I knew it, it was decided. I was going to attend St. Joseph's. No amount of arguing or crying was going to convince my parents to let me go to one of the colleges I was interested in. So I decided to take things into my own hands.

I planned it all very carefully. Skipping breakfast and lunch had been hard at first, but I got used to the hollow feeling in my stomach, and I even grew to like it: It made me feel more in control. The summer's busy social calendar kept my parents preoccupied at night, so dinner often consisted of an apple or yogurt. I was amazed at how many compliments I received for losing weight, despite the fact that my ribs were showing (a fact I tried to keep hidden by wearing layers of tank tops).

A week before I was supposed to leave for St. Joseph's, the critical moment arrived: It was time for my physical. When the nurse weighed me and discovered I was down to ninety-five pounds—a twenty-pound weight loss since last fall—I was counting on the doctor to sound the alarm. Maybe then someone would listen to me!

My plan worked. The doctor couldn't believe how much weight I had lost. She asked me all kinds of questions about how much I was eating and exercising and recommended that I have some blood work done. She said she was very concerned I had an eating disorder.

When my mom told her I was supposed to leave for college the next week, she raised her eyebrows and said, "I don't think Sally should be going anywhere right now. Her health is at risk. She needs intensive outpatient treatment with a therapist and a dietitian to get this eating disorder under control. After I reevaluate her and see that she has gained most of her weight back, *then* you can consider sending her off to college. But you need to realize, that could be months from now."

My mom was stunned. I had made my point. Someone was finally listening.

POINTS TO PONDER

In the above scenario, Sally's sense of self was very much compromised. Her mother had a strong desire to be respected, accepted, and admired by others—something we can all relate to. Unfortunately, this strong desire was expressed in a problematic way. Because she saw her family—and particularly, her daughter—as a reflection on herself, Sally's mother felt she had to control how her daughter was perceived, and therefore had to control many important aspects of her daughter's life. This in turn affected Sally's ability to develop normally and become her own person, an individual separate from her parents.

Sally turned to her eating disorder as a way to gain control of her life and to force her parents to listen to her. Starving her body of needed calories and nutrients also may have provided a way to numb the anger and frustration she felt. Thus, she developed a dependence on her eating disorder to fill a void in her life.

Initially, Sally showed some very healthy responses to this situation. First of all, she showed a desire to break out of the appearance-oriented mold in which she had grown up, and she wanted to do her own thing by finding a job. Second, she showed signs of standing up for herself by arguing with her parents about where they wanted to send her to college. However, when her arguments were disregarded, she felt powerless to have any say in her own future. In an effort to be heard and to assert herself, Sally developed an eating disorder.

Sally yearned for purpose and meaning in her life, for sincere and honest relationships. She found this in her summer job. Miss Emma showed her how to relate to the children in ways she had never experienced before—openly and without pretense, expecting nothing in return. Perhaps if she had shared how great working made her feel, her parents might have been able to validate her feelings and be more supportive. Unfortunately, no one was talking—no one was asking questions or sharing what they were thinking or feeling. This lack of open communication forced Sally to withdraw and find something to fill the empty space in her life. The eating disorder provided a way to both numb her strong feelings and to avoid attending a college she loathed.

Sally's parents apparently had enough money to pay for her college, but her father encouraged her desire to work. This was very beneficial to her developing a sense of pride and independence— qualities she would not have achieved if her dad just handed her a check. Going to work also gave her the opportunity to be out in the world, away from the security of the family home. This in turn allowed her to become more confident and self-assured—which are good life skills, especially if she were to go ahead with her plans to travel abroad.

Parents have a powerful opportunity to recognize their child's uniqueness. In a society so based on outward appearances, a teen's musical, artistic, or scholastic achievements—as well as a caring nature or sense of humor—can easily get overlooked. Placing emphasis on a child's worth as a human being—based on her internal qualities rather than her external characteristics—is an irreplaceable gift. It is, after all, our differences that make us unique and interesting people.

CHANGING THE PATTERN

PARENTS

⁓ Recognize the contribution that your teen's happiness and sense of autonomy will have in her eventual success in life.

⁓ Decide to become a joint architect in your teen's future. Help her to find her voice in determining what happens to her.

⁓ Encourage your teen to make strong, confident, and well-informed decisions for herself.

⁓ Avoid putting too much pressure on your children to excel in ways that *you* think are important.

❧   What does "success" look like to your teen? Ask, and listen to the answer without trying to make it more like your own.

❧   Remember that no child is ever a carbon copy of his or her parent, and try to see the delight and wonder that comes with watching your child become a totally unique individual.

TEENS

❧   Stating the problem and expressing your needs goes a long way toward finding the solution.

❧   Separating and becoming independent is an important part of growing up.

❧   Take responsibility for your words and actions.

❧   Treat your body with care and respect. It depends on you for nourishment.

Scenario 5

THE BLAME GAME

WHEN A PARENT'S INSECURITIES
BECOME PARALYZING

Doubt is a pain too lonely to know that faith is his twin brother.
—Kahlil Gibran

Self-doubt is a double-edged sword: It can be beneficial, leading to increased self-awareness, which in turn prevents impulsive decisions. But more often, it creates ambivalence and prevents necessary action.

For a parent who is enduring an overwhelming major life change, self-doubt can be crippling, as it becomes very difficult to get grounded and confront reality. Minor problems don't get addressed, so they start to mount and worsen, creating a snowball effect, leading to even more self-deprecating thoughts. To protect themselves, adults who are extremely overwhelmed can easily slip into denial about issues that, unconsciously or not, they believe they cannot handle.

Overwhelmed parents, and parents wracked with self-doubt, are prone to being in dangerous denial about a child's eating disorder. For them, it may be too frightening to accept the eating disorder as "real," for the implication (as *they* see it) would mean that they are "horrible parents." But the guilt or shame such parents are afraid of is usually undeserved. The cause of an eating disorder is never that simple and never rests on one person or factor. Nevertheless, .the idea of being responsible for it may feel unbearable. Rather than risking the necessary conversations that could break the ice and create an opening for support, these parents might become psychologically paralyzed and stay silent.

In the following scenario, Ellen, a newly divorced mom, suspects that her fourteen-year-old daughter, Jeannie, is bulimic, but she struggles with reaching out to her because of self-doubt and guilt.

THERE IT IS AGAIN. THE RAP MUSIC FROM THE boom box and the sound of the shower going full blast. Jeannie claims that this nightly after-dinner shower of hers is to help her relax before going to bed. And I can feel every fiber of my body and mind clinging to the hope that she's telling the truth.

But as much as I hate to admit it, my intuition tells me different. Moms have a sixth sense about these things. But then again, you probably wouldn't need to be psychic to know what's really going on. Doesn't it seem obvious? I watch my daughter have three helpings of mashed potatoes and two dishes of ice cream at dinnertime. I hear the muffled sound of the scale ticking as she weighs herself before and after her shower. I see the dark circles under her eyes, and I listen to her ask me whether she's fat every day before she leaves the house for school. I'd probably have to be blind, deaf, and dumb not to notice all these changes, not to sense how much Jeannie has changed. She's lost her sparkle. My little girl—who's always been so effervescent, so full of love and life—is now listless and preoccupied.

Every night during these showers of hers, I start to feel the guilt mounting. Sometimes it even makes me feel nauseated, the whole thing. Where did I go wrong? How have I let Jeannie down? Why did my Jeannie have to be someone with an eating disorder? Did I set a bad example with all the diets I've been experimenting with, trying to drop the ten pounds I gained after my hysterectomy? Is Jeannie trying to drown her feelings about the divorce? Did something terrible happen to my daughter; something she's afraid to tell me about? How did I get to be such a horrible mother?

But then again, maybe it has nothing to do with me. Maybe it's the influence of her friends at school. They're all dieting; I know it. It would be so much easier to blame *Vogue* magazine and Jeannie's friends—especially Sandra, the skinniest fifteen-year-old I've ever seen. Sandra is Jeannie's idol.

Maybe I'm just worrying too much. Maybe this is just a stage girls go through, and there's no need to overreact.

But even when I tried to approach the subject calmly, I got the door slammed in my face. A month ago, I tried to talk to Jeannie about the dangers of dieting at her age. She listened, or pretended to listen, but I could see she was annoyed with me. Finally, I asked her outright one night, after her "shower," if she's been vomiting. Jeannie not only flatly denied it, she seemed horrified. "How could you even think that?" she yelled. "Yuck! I would never do that!" But I'd asked her because I'd found tell-tale signs in the toilet after the showers were over. Seeing the evidence basically forced me to confront her about it. But obviously, that got me nowhere.

What can I possibly do? I feel so helpless. And there's no one to talk with about this—certainly not with Jeannie's father. Since the divorce, he barely even talks to me on the phone. Besides, he'd probably say I was being hysterical again and chastise me for thinking Jeannie could ever do any wrong. As far as he's concerned, she's a perfect angel. I still have a few friends after the divorce, but they're all on diets themselves, and I know that their daughters are dieting too. And what if they judged me for having a bulimic daughter? What if they told their daughters, and then the kids at Jeannie's school found out? That would be a disaster.

My feelings of shame and guilt are literally palpable. I feel as if I'm choking. I need help, but I really don't think there's anyone I can turn to. But at the same time, this feels like so much more than I can handle by myself. Part of me wants to contact a therapist, but my last experience with a shrink was horrible. Dr. Evans completely sided with my husband during the split. What if the therapist blames me for all this? Therapists always seem to think everything's the mother's fault.

But it probably is my fault. It has to be! There's no one else in this house but me and Jeannie. So whose fault could it be but mine? I have to just handle this by myself somehow. It's *my* mess, and I've got to clean it up. And besides, I don't want anyone else to know what I've done to Jeannie. How I don't deserve to be her mother.

POINTS TO PONDER

The actual factors that may have led to Jeannie's eating disorder were not made known in this scenario, but parental guilt and denial were contributing to its continuation. Already affected by the pain of a divorce, Ellen was immobilized by her fear of facing a situation that could make her feel even worse. She was obviously concerned for Jeannie's welfare but couldn't bring herself to confront what she knew was a serious threat to Jeannie's physical and emotional health.

Ellen was obviously struggling with several problems. First of all, she was showing signs of doubt and denial. For even though all evidence indicated that Jeannie was bulimic, Ellen still found herself wondering whether she was just making things up, or whether she was overreacting—even though she was not really reacting at all.

Second, Ellen was overly preoccupied with the fear of being blamed—by herself and by society—for her daughter's eating disorder. She spent a lot of time alternating between 1) feeling shame and guilt about her ability as a mother, and 2) guessing and hoping that someone else might be to blame besides herself.

Even conscientious parents sometimes believe that enough guilt and blame will magically bring about a solution, but they are absolutely wrong. In fact, turning in on oneself is destructive and merely focuses energy on the problem instead of the solution. Although Ellen may not have been able to rid herself immediately of the feelings of guilt, shame, and blame, she needed to emerge from her ambivalence long enough to talk honestly to Jeannie and get her the help she needed.

Granted, it is difficult to be rational and objective when haunted by feelings of guilt, but there was at least one very simple step that Ellen could have taken to empower herself: She could have started to educate herself about eating disorders. By so doing, she would have discovered that eating disorders are influenced by many factors, not by just one person or situation. That discovery alone could have alleviated enough guilt to puncture her paralysis and bring about effective action.

Ellen's lack of confidence in herself was made even more troublesome because of her lack of faith in her own friends and in the therapeutic process—making it more challenging to get the support she needed and deserved in order to help her daughter recover. In addition to educating themselves about eating disorders and addressing their own attitudes about body image and thinness, parents who are overwhelmed need to give themselves permission to seek support from a trusted friend, minister, rabbi, counselor, or family member. Helping a child recover from an eating disorder is extremely stressful, and parents often need as much support as the child.

Also, it would have been beneficial for Ellen to examine her own attitudes toward thinness and dieting. After she gained some clarity about herself, she could have begun to share those thoughts and feelings with Jeannie, and could have encouraged her daughter to talk about her own thoughts and feelings on the subject. Even if Ellen feared that her own attitudes toward food and body image were less than perfect, if she took the risk of sharing them with her daughter, it probably would have made it easier for her daughter to do the same. Ellen, like many parents, was reluctant to divulge her innermost feelings, but if she would have been able to do so, it might have been one of the most powerful factors in Jeannie's recovery. If Jeannie saw that her mother was willing to change, Jeannie might have had an easier time believing that she too could change. Her mother's honesty could have helped Jeannie to see her mother as a real person—a human being, with vulnerabilities and faults—and spurred Jeannie on to become more real as well.

Ellen's half-hearted attempts to talk to Jeannie about her eating disorder fell on deaf ears. Jeannie was extremely defensive, in part because an eating disorder feels like such an intensely private thing, but also because she knew her mom would be terribly upset if she knew the truth. To counter Jeannie's defensiveness, the most effective language Ellen could have used would have been words that created a safe place for Jeannie to talk, and not words of stark confrontation. How could Ellen have conveyed these messages? Perhaps by saying something similar to this: "Jeannie, it really is safe to tell me the truth. I can handle whatever you tell me. We will find a solution together. I love you and want you to be happy. I am not blaming either of us." Each parent in a similar situation will have her or his own words, but a straightforward, confident, loving, and accepting approach is powerful and effective.

CHANGING THE PATTERN

PARENTS

⬱   Instead of taking on guilt for causing the problem, take on responsibility for your role in the recovery.

⬱   Get the information and help you need and deserve. Eating-disorder professionals have no interest in judging or blaming—only in sharing insight, giving support, and assisting in the recovery process.

⬱   Use direct, loving, accepting messages when confronting your teen about an eating disorder.

❧ When talking to your teen, refer to the eating disorder as "our problem," not "your problem." This inclusive approach is less alienating for the teen.

TEENS

❧ If a parent asks you directly about your eating disorder, tell the truth. Hiding your secret will only make it worse.

❧ Don't take on guilt, and don't assign guilt to your parents. Your eating disorder is no one's fault. However, everyone plays a vital role in the recovery process.

❧ Seek a therapist to help you and your parents. A therapist can encourage you to reclaim your healthy self and help your parents to support your recovery. There are times when we cannot fix a problem alone.

❧ Continue your honest conversations with your parents as you recover. Open communication will hasten your recovery and build closeness with those who are supporting you.

Scenario 6

HIDING OUT WITH THE SKELETONS

WHEN PARENTS SUFFER
FROM ADDICTION

The task ahead of us is never as great as the power behind us.
—Alcoholics Anonymous

Alcohol and drug addiction is rampant in our society. Causes are hard to pinpoint, but contributing factors include genetic predisposition, social influences, and psychological factors. Addiction does not mean that the sufferer is "bad" or "weak," but rather is in the grip of a progressive disease that affects every member of his or her family. Adults who are trying unsuccessfully to juggle multiple roles and responsibilities can turn to substances to numb the pressures of life, or to substitute for the lack of real emotional connections with others.

Spouses and children are affected adversely when adults who struggle with substance abuse or dependence remain in denial and don't seek the help they need. On some level, teens always sense when there is a secret in the family. They worry about themselves and their parents if there is an unspoken understanding that an addictive behavior can't be discussed. Moreover, the silence surrounding the addiction—and the taboo about bringing it out in the open—causes teens to question their own sense of reality. Confusion sets in about what is real, and how they should cope with problems. When alcoholism clouds the close bond they had with their parents, they experience loss of relationship and turn to other forms of comfort. Because the teens have learned, by example, the behavior of using a substance or action (such as bingeing) to numb their pain and loneliness, they may turn to that dysfunctional response as well.

In the following scenario, thirteen-year-old Lindsey takes refuge from her parents' denial and unhappiness by retreating to her closet and creating a secret ritual of bingeing and cutting.

I HAVE A RITUAL. A CEREMONY. AND IT'S

secret. No one in my family knows. No one in my family notices. But this is what I do:

I go into my walk-in closet, turn on the light, and shut the door. I reach up and get the sewing needle. It is carefully hidden, stashed away on the top shelf, behind my old backpack. Then, sitting on the floor in my closet, I take a deep breath and began to carve the letter L, for Lindsey, on my forearm, watching the crimson blood ooze its way out of the perfectly etched lines. My body goes limp, and my mind goes numb, and I feel better with every movement of the needle. Once I feel more relaxed, I reach into the box in the back of the closet and get out the big bag of M&Ms I always keep there. And then I eat them, as many as I can possibly eat.

I can completely relax in there, because I'm not worried about ever being caught. My brother is never home, even on school nights. He's always out cruising with his friends. Mom and Dad are always home, but they're always oblivious, sitting at the kitchen table, drinking vodka from their coffee cups. Do they think I'm buying it when they say they're drinking coffee? Tina and Susan said vodka doesn't have an odor, and that's why they drink it, but they're wrong: Every morning, when I wash the dishes from last night while everyone is still sleeping, I can smell the sharp odor of alcohol in the coffee cups.

Most times when I get home from school, Mom is sipping from her mug and watching *Dr. Phil*. I can always tell when she's been drinking vodka instead of coffee, because she gets mad at me about something stupid, like putting my books down on the stairs instead of the table—stuff she would never yell about if she weren't drinking. And then, even more ridiculous, she starts yelling that she's going to have Dad swat my bottom when he gets home, to teach me a lesson about my lazy, sloppy habits. How old do they think I am?

Dad must think it's ridiculous too, because he just tells me to pretend to cry so Mom thinks he's spanking me. And Mom never bothers to check, because she's glued to the TV and her cup of so-called coffee. Sometimes I wonder whether she knows the truth but just doesn't want to deal with it. I feel bad about being dishonest with her. But Dad doesn't seem to care. He hides other things from Mom too, like his relationship with Mrs. Peters. He introduced me to Mrs. Peters a few times, and asked that I not tell Mom. It makes me feel awful.

And when I feel like that, I go to the closet to start my ritual. It's not perfect, but it helps—a lot. Even though I'm all the way upstairs, in my closet with the door shut, I can still hear Mom and Dad when they're screaming at each other in the kitchen, calling each other lousy parents and slamming pots and pans around. But at least in the closet the sounds are muffled. And at least the needle and the chocolate make me not care so much about any of it. I can sit there for hours, daydreaming about being thin and famous, like the Hollywood Stars. But I'm not delusional—I know even they don't have perfect lives. It can't be easy to have people following you all the time and wanting your autograph. When they are sad, I bet they sit in their closets full of beautiful clothes and eat chocolate like I do. I bet some of them cut themselves too.

No one knows about my parents and my cutting and bingeing except my best friend, Jana. Even though I do a good job of hiding my scars and my feelings, Jana knows me way too well, and we are way too close, for her not to notice. Jana really wants to tell her mom and swears that her mom will only help, but I told her I would *kill* her if she did that. I would be horrified if anyone else knew about this, and I couldn't stand the thought of Jana's mom judging my parents.

The other day, though, Jana asked me a really good question—one I'd never thought of before: "What does your brother think about your parents' drinking?" I honestly didn't know. I'm not that close to him, but part of me knows that he is never home because life at our house is so miserable. Jana is such a great friend and so smart to ask me that. She said, "Maybe you can ask him about it. It might be easier to talk to your parents about this if your brother is with you. And remember, I am here to help, and my mom would be very understanding if I told her. My grandpa was an alcoholic, so she would understand what it's like for you—but she also knows that judging or accusing your parents is not going to help."

She made me promise to at least talk to my brother, and I said I would, but I don't know. Maybe I'm not ready to take that step yet. And even if my brother joined me, the thought of confronting my parents about their drinking is so scary. I'm not even sure what would happen. Would they change the subject? Would they freak out?

Maybe my brother would have some answers. But it seems so weird to talk to him about something so intense. We're not close . . . but we *used* to be. He is older though, and more experienced. Even if we don't talk to Mom and Dad about their drinking, maybe I won't feel so alone if I talk with him about it. I don't know. I'm just so scared. It feels like there's a ticking time bomb in this house, and I have no idea how to defuse it.

POINTS TO PONDER

In this scenario, Lindsey was on her way to becoming a compulsive overeater, or closet eater, which leads to low self-esteem, social isolation, shame, depression, and obesity. The disordered eating she had already developed could have eventually led to bulimia or anorexia.

Lindsey's family dynamics were characterized by addiction, open conflict, and double binds (which occur when someone is given conflicting messages). These family dynamics are much more common for compulsive overeaters and teens with bulimia than for teens with anorexia. Bulimia is a chaotic pattern that tends to develop in families that have open conflict, disorganized eating, and addictive behavior. Anorexic families are more apt to avoid conflict and to have high expectations for perfect behavior. Secrets can be common in both. To cope with the chaos, Lindsey developed a pattern of cutting herself in addition to overeating. Together, these behaviors became a numbing ritual. The cutting created physical pain, which worked to distract her from her emotional pain, while the eating numbed her feelings and comforted her.

It may also be that the cutting was a response to the guilt she felt for colluding with her dad to deceive her mother. At the same time, it was a way to take out, on herself, the uncomfortable anger she must have felt toward both of her parents for putting her in an impossible double bind.

Sadly, all of these methods of coping were going on without her parents' knowledge, because they were caught up in their own addictions. Lindsey was virtually alone in trying to get her needs for love and attention met in the only ways she knew how. Her food stash became her source of nurturing. When she ate and cut, she escaped into a fantasy world, where she could identify with glamorous people who seemed romantic to her. She suspected that the stars she idolized had their own secret rituals of cutting and bingeing simply because their lives couldn't be perfect either. It soothed her to think that they were often sad and lonely, just as she was. In addition, identifying with them created an imaginary emotional bond that she desperately needed and wasn't feeling with her parents. Her sadness was intensified, because she remembered when her parents had been there for her, and she longed for that closeness again. She heard the drunken sounds from the kitchen, but they were muffled and forgotten when she was bingeing and cutting.

If Lindsey had been able to tell her parents that she was lonely and desperate for their attention, and if they could have heard her and responded, she would not have needed the refuge of her closet and the cutting behavior. If she could have penetrated their alcoholic fog, she could have received support for the problems every teenager deals with. If her father had not expected her to keep the secret about his involvement with Mrs. Peters, she wouldn't feel the double bind for which she, at her age, had no coping mechanisms. Lindsey actually had no consistent parenting and was attempting to take care of herself in the only way she could create for herself.

Teens are extremely vulnerable to adverse effects of parental drinking, because they are already dealing with the pressures of grades, dating, developing an identity, and trying to be accepted. If parents are struggling with addictions, teens can feel lost and alone as they face these new pressures. When parents are in an unconscious state, they can't be available for the support and guidance so needed by their children during this crucial stage in their development.

Sadly, such a family atmosphere is fertile ground for the development of an eating disorder, as well as other harmful behaviors, such as cutting. Addicted parents may miss important warning signs of an impending eating disorder, because the alcohol numbs them to what their children feel and need. Parental denial of the effect their addiction is having on their children is a threat to the health and happiness of everyone in the family. Parents who are naturally caring and attentive can become distracted when their use of alcohol reaches the level of an addiction, and their children miss out on the nurturing that their parents may have provided prior to the onset of their addiction.

In the best of all worlds, having to address the crisis of a child's eating disorder becomes a vehicle for the parents to face their own addictions. In fact, children sometimes unconsciously develop a problem like this, secretly hoping that their parents will also get help. Sadly, addicted parents can sometimes have difficulty facing their roles in the teen's recovery, regardless of counseling or their teen's need. In this case, all is not lost for the teen: A caring friend, teacher, or neighbor can offer the support necessary for healing to begin. Reaching out to a trusted adult other than a parent may feel like betrayal, but taking that step may help teens like Lindsey feel supported enough to talk to their parents about how their drinking affects them. Teens should also enlist a sibling's support and help as they consider breaking the silence and confronting their parents. At a young age, it is scary to confront, all by yourself, a secret that has ruled the family and prevented honest communication.

Even when a family is crippled by alcoholism or other addictions, there are avenues for help for the teen who is affected. Teachers, school counselors, ministers or rabbis, and other trusted adults in the teen's life can offer counsel and guidance. Self-help groups such as Al-Anon and Alateen are available, and many schools have counseling groups for kids. Parents will often agree to take their teens to therapy for the child's surface problem, and then the therapist can help to intervene in the family system where addiction is the issue. If a teen like Lindsey reaches out to someone, the cycle of recovery can begin.

CHANGING THE PATTERN

PARENTS

🙥 If your son or daughter is developing problems with binge eating or another eating disorder, and you are struggling with your own addiction, face your problem head on, and go for help. Your children's physical and emotional health, as well as yours, is at stake.

🙥 If your teenager courageously asks you to face your own drinking or drug problem—one that causes pain in his or her life—try to listen and not hide. Many eating disorders have been derailed midstream because parents began to listen without becoming defensive.

🙥 Congratulate yourself for deciding to come out of your own closet of addictive behavior, and for having the courage to change a pattern that is affecting the entire family.

TEENS

🙥 As hard as it may be, try to tell your parents how you feel about any habits or addictions they have that bother you. To increase the chance that they will listen, describe *your* feelings, without pointing a finger at them.

🙥 If you feel your parents will not listen to your concerns, find an adult you trust, and share your feelings. It could be a counselor at school, a neighbor, or a relative who cares about you.

☙ Your eating disorder may be trying to speak for you. When you dare to use your voice to tell your parents how their behavior is affecting you, you have launched your recovery process.

☙ Helping your parents face the truth is never a betrayal, even though it can feel that way. Truth-telling brings healing and recovery.

SUPPLEMENTARY READING AND RESOURCES

FOR PARENTS

When Your Child Is Cutting: A Parent's Guide to Helping Children Overcome Self-Injury, by Merry E. McVey-Woble, PhD, Sony Khemlani-Patel, PhD, and Fugen Neziroglu, PhD

FOR TEENS

For Teenagers Living with a Parent Who Abuses Alcohol/Drugs, by Edith Lynn Hornik-Beer

Also, for more information for teens with a parent addicted to alcohol, contact: **Al-Anon/Alateen,** www.al-anon.alateen.org, 1-800-4AL-ANON (1-800-425-2666)

Scenario 7

TOO COOL FOR SCHOOL

WHEN THE RULES OF FRIENDSHIP

SUDDENLY CHANGE

The young always have the same problem: how to rebel and conform at the same time. They have now solved this by defying their parents and copying one another.

—Quentin Crisp

The transition from elementary school to middle school can be a mine field for girls. Not only are they overwhelmed with pressures to look pretty, dress "right," and have the perfect body, but they are also expected to fit in with the popular crowd and to be smart— but not *too* smart. Add to that the fact that they are moving from a smaller, familiar campus to a much larger, unfamiliar one; and are shifting from having one or two teachers who knew them well, to five or six teachers whose personalities and academic demands may be very different. Suddenly, and often without warning, the rules have changed. This can be very intimidating and unsettling to a young adolescent who lacks the ability to understand what's going on and the experience to articulate her feelings and fears, or to ask questions.

In the following scenario, eleven-year-old Becky experiences a rude awakening about friendship, popularity, and being smart when she starts middle school.

I COULDN'T WAIT TO START SIXTH GRADE

and go to Valley View Middle School. Finally I would be one of the big kids. Mom and Dad always kidded me about wanting to grow up too fast. But I was sick of being in elementary school, stuck with all the kindergarteners and first graders! At Valley View, I'd get my own locker, and I'd get to change classrooms and teachers every period. It sounded really fun.

I'll admit it though: It *was* nice to be in the highest grade last year. Everybody looks up to you when you're the oldest. My teacher, Ms. P, had asked me at the beginning of the school year if I wanted to tutor some of the younger students in math. She probably could tell I was starting to get bored. Math was really easy for me, and it seemed like I was so far ahead of everyone else in my class. Tutoring gave me a new challenge, and I had a ton of fun doing it. Jamie, a first-grader, was my favorite kid to tutor. He even told me how much fun I made learning how to add and subtract. I started thinking that maybe I'd be a teacher when I grew up.

Luckily, all my best friends were also going to Valley View, so I wasn't worried about having to start from scratch. That would have been horrible, especially after all the work I put into being popular. But it didn't take me long to realize that things are somehow different now. Even my friends are acting strange. They seem like different people all of a sudden, and I don't understand why. For example, yesterday, in math class, when I raised my hand to answer a question, I saw Billy Davis—the hottest guy in school—roll his eyes, and I heard him mumble something under his breath. He was making fun of me for speaking up in class. I thought I was going to die.

That's when it hit me: Ever since I started at Valley View, my friends have been kind of teasing me and making snide remarks about me, about how I'm too smart. It seems all they want to talk about these days are boys, being fat, and what new diet they are trying. I just don't get it anymore! Even Mary and Kathy are saying they're fat, but they are really skinny! Sarah is all of a sudden the cool girl in our group, ever since she announced to everyone that she had already lost six pounds. I told my mom that I was worried about my friends, because a lot of them are not eating lunch anymore so that they will lose weight. She sighed and said, "I'm so glad you're not doing those crazy things." But what about my friends? I guess she wasn't worried, so maybe I shouldn't be either. Still, I wanted to tell her more about it, like about how I feel bad sitting at our table at lunch. Now my friends play this new game and whisper back and forth, laughing and making fun of every girl's body as she goes through the cafeteria line. Girls they don't even know!

Today, when I got home from school, I ran upstairs and stared at myself in the closet mirror. I was terrified. What were they saying about *me?* They must think I look like a moose! I felt panic setting in. If I don't go on a diet and lose weight, my friends won't like me anymore. They'll even start to make fun of me. I know I can do whatever I set my mind to, that's what Mom and Dad always say. So from now on, no breakfast or lunch, and just a little food at dinner. And no more raising my hand in class, that's for sure! And maybe my homework doesn't need to be done every single day. Other kids get away with not doing their homework all the time. If this is what it takes to fit in, then I will make it work.

POINTS TO PONDER

In this scenario, Becky did not yet have an eating disorder, but she seemed well on her way to developing one. Like many girls her age, Becky placed a high value on being popular, and unfortunately, the girls she admired were suddenly "changing the rules" on her. With her achievement-oriented personality, her desire to be popular, and the insecurities that naturally come with being in middle school, Becky was ready to do whatever it took to maintain her status among her friends—even if that meant becoming a poor student and forcing herself to diet and lose weight.

Becky is the "easy" kid—the one parents don't worry about because she excels in school, has a good group of friends, and in general seems happy and content. Unfortunately, parents of this kind of teen can be caught off guard. It's possible for them to be unaware of their teen's cry for help, because she always seems to be able to handle things well. When Becky's world began to fall apart, she tried to talk to her mom but was quickly dismissed, since her mom thought her daughter was handling the situation. Without thinking there might be anything more to Becky's concerns, she was just relieved that her daughter wasn't "doing those crazy things." By asking a few simple questions, Becky's mom may have been able to pick up on her worry about her own weight, and would have been able to give her the support she needed.

Early adolescent minds are just beginning to shift from concrete thinking (based on objects, such as people, places, or things) to abstract thinking (ideas, principles, and symbols). Until they have fully made the transition into being able to think abstractly, they may still see the world in black-and-white terms, missing shades of gray. To young teenagers, their bodies and food are very concrete and familiar in a world where new ideas and challenges may seem pretty frightening. It makes sense that they would turn to the concrete world of body and food to cope with their strong emotions and feelings of insecurity. Faced with the idea that she might lose her friends or that they might think she was fat, Becky turned to the only thing she knew she had control over—her eating and her weight.

Puberty, which occurs in the middle-school years, is a difficult time for both children and parents. For teens, this is a time of tremendous physical and emotional change. Their bodies are changing, their hormones are raging, and they have an increased awareness of the world around them. Their peers become all important, and parents are suddenly looked at as if they live on another planet.

Parents all want their children to mature into well-adjusted, healthy adults. But they can no longer protect their teens from peer pressures and society's influences. Despite the fact that teens often give us the impression that what parents think isn't important, in many cases, they actually *do* care—it just isn't cool to show it. Even though teens often seem unwilling to talk to parents about what is happening at school or with their friends, parents can still be there to listen and provide a sounding board for them when they *do* choose to share their concerns or experiences.

Busy lives and responsibilities often hinder us from this important interaction. But there are ways around this. Let's say a teen comes to a parent with a concern, but what the parent is doing simply can't be put off. The parent can say, "Wow, you sound really worried about that. Let's sit down and talk in fifteen minutes." It's a simple reaction, but instead of feeling dismissed, the teen will understand he or she is being heard and that his or her concerns are important. Another way for parents to ensure they are involved with their teens' emotional lives and available to listen is to schedule time every two weeks for checking in. Perhaps, if the family budget allows, this meeting could take place over a meal at the teen's favorite restaurant. These types of meetings not only create a regular, natural-feeling atmosphere of sharing thoughts and feelings, but they also encourage a healthy enjoyment of the teen's favorite foods. If you think your teen may be concerned about having such talks in public, consider getting his or her favorite takeout, or have a "pizza night."

Adolescence is the time when children begin to form their own value systems and to make choices that may very well determine their future. They need their parents to be involved and available to them. Their physical needs may not be as great as they were in early childhood, but their emotional needs require constant monitoring.

CHANGING THE PATTERN

PARENTS

❧ Try to have a regular heart-to-heart talk with your teen during times of major changes. It is particularly important to be in touch with your teen when he or she is changing schools.

❧ Be aware of any subtle comments your teen makes and the hidden messages he or she is trying to convey.

❧ Ask your teen whether his or her performance at school feels different or judged, and have an open conversation with them about how to make and keep friends without compromising their schoolwork or their own personalities.

❧ Keep your teen away from dieting at all costs. Diets are dangerous and are considered a risk factor in the development of eating disorders. Instead, help your adolescent learn balance, variety, and moderation in eating, and encourage a healthy level of daily activity.

❧ Encourage your teen to value what is best in themselves and others. Show them by example that it is what's inside that counts.

TEENS

❧ Choose your friends wisely; they will influence who you will become.

❧ Remember that restricting calories doesn't just compromise your health—it can also keep you from reaching your full height.

❧ Keep in mind that kids who tease are feeling uncomfortable and insecure with themselves. If you can be understanding of that, their words won't hurt so much.

❧ Being physically active helps you feel and look your best. Find physical activities that you enjoy. It's also a great way to meet new friends!

Scenario 8

SO LITTLE TIME

WHEN KIDS ARE OVERBOOKED

A man must be master of his hours and days, not their servant.
—William Frederick Book

Today's children are often overscheduled. Parents also may feel overscheduled because of the pressures of work, and they may not have enough time to "just be" with their kids. Children grow up quickly, especially in today's world. That is why it is vitally important for parents and children to communicate and stay connected about what each family member needs. Parents are the most important teachers and the greatest support system for their kids. When children or parents are overcommitted, their relationships and sense of self can be damaged. Taking the time to set priorities and schedule downtime might at first seem strange, but both children and parents thrive in this kind of environment.

Scheduling regular family meals and snacks can help bring busy families together and can prevent eating problems. Disordered eating, as opposed to an eating disorder, refers to troublesome eating behaviors that may include dieting, bingeing, or purging, but which generally occur less frequently or are less severe than those of an eating disorder. Disordered eating can be changes in eating patterns that occur in response to stress, an illness, personal appearance, or an athletic competition.

In the following scenario, fourteen-year-old Vicky and her younger brother, Kyle, are constantly in fourth gear because their parents want them to have every advantage.

THE DOOR OF THE VAN SLAMMED SHUT, AND

Mom jumped into the driver's seat, screaming, "Buckle your seat belts!" The tires squealed as she backed the car out of the driveway and raced down the street. Kyle and I looked at each other, thinking, "This is crazy." But what could we do? What could we say?

Mom had come home from work late that day, and I was already late for my ballet lesson. Kyle could still make it on time for soccer practice—if we were lucky and made all the green lights.

Everything is so hectic at our house, but Kyle and I are pretty much used to it. Both of us have music lessons on

Mondays and French and karate lessons on Wednesdays. Kyle has soccer practice on Tuesdays and Thursdays, and I have ballet class at the same time. Friday is our only day off, because Kyle plays soccer on Saturdays, and we try to go to church on Sundays—if we're not all too worn out. But we usually are.

Mom and Dad think it's important for us to take advantage of every opportunity "while we are still young." They don't want us to miss out on anything worthwhile. I'm not so sure I feel the same way. I really like everything I'm involved in, and I think Kyle does too, but it is getting harder and harder to keep up with school and all my lessons. I never have any time to just hang with my friends or go to a movie, because Kyle, my mom, and I are always on the road to the next activity. Dad can hardly ever join us because of work, so it seems like we never see him.

Life has been crazy since Mom and Dad decided to bite the bullet three years ago: They used up all their savings to build their dream house. And to help keep us afloat, Mom went back to work.

At first, we were all really excited about our huge new house. Kyle and Dad were especially excited about kicking a ball around the huge yard and shooting hoops in the basketball court we installed. But they never have any time to do that anymore. I was really excited about my new big bedroom, but I hate the fact that Mom is never there when I get home from school. Even though I'm not happy about the way things are, I don't want to complain to Mom and Dad. They have sacrificed so much. It would seem selfish of me to complain about everything they are trying to do for us.

Also, now I have to watch over Kyle until Mom gets home from work. Kyle's okay as brothers go, but sometimes he doesn't come right home from school like he's supposed to, and since I'm the one who's responsible, I get really worried. I can't blame him for not coming right home though. Who wants to come home to a big empty house? Just because I'm old enough to be home alone doesn't mean I like it. I miss talking to Mom after school. I miss how she used to be actually interested in how my day went. Now the only time Mom talks to me is when she's yelling at me to hurry up.

The only thing that keeps me occupied while I'm home alone, waiting for everyone to show up, is eating. But I'm worried, because I weighed myself the other day, and I've gained a few pounds—just what I needed! Now, I'm going to have to figure out a way to lose it. That's going to be really hard, because I'm starving when I get home from school. Oh, yeah, that's the other thing. Mom never has time to pack a lunch for Kyle and me anymore, so we have to do it ourselves. I usually don't get up early enough, so I just throw a yogurt or granola bar in my backpack as I run out the door to the bus. Now this stupid weight-gain thing. I don't know what I'm going to do.

Plus, I'm worried about Mom and Dad. They both seem so stressed out lately. Mom is always complaining about how much weight she is gaining and how fat she looks, but she never takes time to exercise or do anything about it because she's too busy. I'd love to ask her help with my weight problem, but she's obviously not doing too well herself, and I don't want to worry her. I've noticed that Dad is starting to have a drink every night to relax, and it seems like the two of them hardly ever talk to each other anymore. By the time they get home from work and are done chauffeuring me and Kyle everywhere, all they seem to want to do is fall on the couch and watch TV. Even Kyle has noticed. Yesterday he asked, "Vicky, can you even remember the last time we sat down for dinner as a family and Mom actually cooked something instead of heating up a frozen pizza or ordering takeout?"

Why in the world did we buy such a nice house when we are never home to enjoy it?

POINTS TO PONDER

In today's world, there is so much competition for children to be good at everything—be it sports, academics, music, or other creative arts. There is also pressure early on for them to get into the best schools—not just colleges, but also high schools, and now, even preschools. Is it any wonder that conscientious parents sometimes think that the more involved their children are, the more opportunities they will have? But the fact is that overscheduling can make parents fall out of touch with their children's emotional lives. In this scenario, Vicky and Kyle were clearly overbooked and overstressed.

Vicky was overwhelmed by the commitments and time constraints on her life. She used food as an outlet for all the pressure she was under. She also found some relief about her concerns for her mom and dad through eating. Stress can create changes in our eating behaviors. Some of us eat more, and some of us eat less in response to emotions. We might also miss a meal now and then when we are on the run, or eat too much or too little at meals when we are preoccupied.

What distinguishes "disordered eating" from occasional overeating or skipping meals is the purpose and consistency behind the behavior, and whether or not the individuals can maintain a sense of control or free choice with regard to their eating behaviors. Vicky was clearly in danger of becoming more compulsive about her food choices and more limited in what and how much she would allow herself to eat, since it was meeting an emotional need. By definition, an eating disorder is a misuse of food to resolve emotional problems.

Although Vicky did not, as yet, have a full blown eating disorder, it can be a slippery slope for young people who have turned to food to resolve some inner conflict or to meet an emotional need. Had Vicky's parents been able to be more present, and less burdened by the financial strain the new house had placed on them, they may have been more aware of Vicky's new eating patterns and better able to help turn things around before it was too late. The good news is that disordered eating does not usually develop into a clinical eating disorder, particularly if there is early recognition and effective intervention. However, if disordered eating becomes sustained or begins to interfere with everyday activities, it may require professional evaluation.

All loving parents want their children to "have it all." But providing them with every opportunity is not beneficial when it means sacrificing their kids' mental and emotional health, and when it means there is no longer any time to enjoy each other's company. By placing work and possessions ahead of family time and self-care, a troublesome message is being sent. Allowing downtime—for parents and children alike—is extremely important. Downtime creates an atmosphere in which people have the capacity to listen and the mental space to hear one another, and as a result, an environment is created in which communication thrives.

In a September 10, 2004 *Seattle Post-Intelligencer* article, Anthony B. Robinson addressed the subject of this scenario, saying, "Hyper-parenting skews the relationship of parents and children, as children are turned into products and performers and parents into managers and handlers." He went on to explain how important—but tricky—it is for parents to find the right balance between two kinds of love: accepting love and transforming love. Accepting love *affirms* the "being" of a child and lets him "be," while transforming love *seeks* his well-being and prods his growth. Hyper-parenting is an excess of the latter and a deficiency of the former.

Parents can and should offer challenges and opportunities to their children, but taking the responsibility to also help them learn healthy lifestyle patterns, which promote balance and moderation, is key. This will result in happier and better-adjusted children, in addition to promoting healthier relationships within the family system.

CHANGING THE PATTERN

PARENTS

❧ Listen carefully if your child is complaining of not wanting to participate in a game or practice the piano. They may be overbooked or feeling overwhelmed, and may not know how to tell you. They could also be afraid they will disappoint you.

❧ Evaluate priorities, remembering to balance material desires with the needs of the family members.

❧ Instead of filling your children's free time with sports and other activities outside the family, consider scheduling a game night. A quick game of basketball or board games as a family are good ways to strengthen bonds between parents and children.

❧ Make time for quality time. Schedule romantic dinner dates with your mate and special time with each child.

❧ Remember that it's okay—perfectly healthy and natural—to veg out and do nothing sometimes. Everyone needs relaxation, alone time, and time to enjoy friends and family.

TEENS

❧ If you are persistently feeling anxious or depressed, or are having trouble sleeping, let your parents know. These can be signs of too much stress or being involved in too many activities. How much a person can handle is different for everyone. Learn and honor what is right for you.

❧ Tell your parents that having some downtime allows you to explore who you are and who you want to become. It also allows you to spend time with friends and family.

❧ Remember: The best way to maintain a healthy weight is to eat at least three meals a day consisting of all the food groups, plus one to three healthy snacks.

SUPPLEMENTARY READING:

FOR PARENTS

The Over-Scheduled Child: Avoiding the Hyper-Parenting Trap, by Alvin Rosenfeld and Nicole Wise

Scenario 9

TREAD SOFTLY . . .

WHEN A TEEN HAS A
SENSITIVE TEMPERAMENT

*I was thinking that I might fly today / Just to disprove all
the things you say / Please be careful with me / I'm sensitive,
and I'd like to stay that way.*

—Jewel

Sensitivity is both a gift and a burden. Noticing what others feel,
and what is going on inside oneself, can be an asset and can bring
about caring behavior and self-awareness. On the other hand,
experiencing life at this depth can create strong reactions to what
others think, especially when criticism is perceived.

Some people seem to be born with a sensitive temperament,
and others acquire it at an early age. Unfortunately, sensitivity
often provides fertile ground for the development of compulsive
behaviors such as eating disorders, because reacting negatively to

the opinions of others can seem overwhelming and can affect self-esteem. Starving, or bingeing and purging, can temporarily numb the sting of hurt feelings or provide a false sense of security when the world seems harsh and judging.

Many sensitive girls find themselves drawn to dance and ballet, activities that are also known for their focus on a particular body shape and size. As puberty approaches, these young female dancers reach a critical point when their bodies' natural changes are scrutinized in terms of the kind of future they may have as dancers. If negative attention is brought to their body shape or size at this crucial stage, they can turn to an eating disorder to bring about what they think is a remedy. And oftentimes dance instructors are not aware of the power they have to contribute to self-consciousness in a young girl who is already sensitive and needs affirmation and reassurance, not criticism.

In the following scenario, thirteen-year-old Anne has an understandable reaction to words that are intended to motivate but actually serve as a trigger to her eating-disordered behavior.

FROM ACROSS THE DANCE FLOOR, I SAW MS.

White coming toward me, and I froze in the middle of my stretch. My heart thumped under my leotard, and all of her previous comments—about the "importance of form" and how a ballerina has to be "light as a feather"—rushed into my mind. I noted her tight jaw, her frozen expression, and her determined step. *This is it,* I told myself. For months, I'd been trying to deny the truth: I've gotten too big to do this. But all that denial crumbled in a nanosecond.

Mom and Dad have told me a million times that I'm not fat. But if I'm going to be a real ballet dancer, I have to be thin—it's the only way. I know I'm only thirteen and I haven't stopped growing, but I have carefully studied some of the older girls' bodies, and they all look willowy and graceful.

I stared at the floor, too scared to look up, but I could feel her critical eyes on me, and I could imagine all the curious and pitying looks from the other students. Then I remembered what Mom and Dad said about how I tend to worry too much, and how I think that other people are always judging me, but that it's probably not true. *Maybe the other students aren't staring at me,* I thought. *Maybe they are just stretching like I am.* Still, I was too scared to look. If they *were* staring at me, it would be like a nightmare.

Mom and Dad keep reminding me that I shouldn't be comparing myself to them, especially since I'm the youngest dancer in the class. Mom used to dance when she was young, and she said that she knows from experience: A couple of years is a big difference at my age. She said I have to be patient; that it will be a while before I am as accomplished as the others.

But Ms. White was standing over me, and I was praying for her to be distracted by something, or for her to be called away by a phone call. But I wasn't so lucky. I could feel my face go red, and I braced myself for what was coming.

"Anne," said Ms. White. "If you don't get rid of *this,* you will never qualify to be a dancer in my troupe." Her finger traced an imaginary line slowly and precisely across my abdomen. The humiliation felt like a rush of ice water through my blood, and with a spurt of determination I'd never experienced before, I looked right into her eyes.

"Thank you, Ms. White." I said. "You will never have to mention this again."

I suffered through the last twenty minutes of my dance class. I couldn't remember a time when I felt so bad about myself. I wanted the floor to swallow me up and take me away. I looked at no one, and no one talked to me. They had probably heard what Ms. White said and didn't want it to happen to them.

Everything was too confusing. Who was right? Ms. White or my parents? I could feel the battle going on inside of me. *Am I okay the way I am, or do I need to be smaller so I can be the kind of dancer Ms. White wants in her troupe?* I was more miserable than I had ever been. I had always wanted to go to New York and become a ballet star. None of that could happen now unless I majorly changed how my body looked. I thought there still might be a chance—if I figured out how to diet. It was worth a try at least. I could at least try to lose weight fast and follow my dream of being a famous dancer. I would show Ms. White that I could do it.

It seemed like forever before my mother appeared at the door to give me a ride home. She said something about how quiet I was but then didn't ask me anything else. I was too hurt and confused to explain to her what had happened. And I was afraid that she would be disappointed in me. I wanted her to notice how bad I felt, but she was talking on and on about how she needed to go to the supermarket and get something for dinner before Dad got home. I wasn't sure it was safe to tell her I had decided to lose weight.

The next day I talked to my friend Katie about how to lose weight. She had started a diet about a month before and lost a ton of weight. Talking to her really helped me. She told me she became a vegetarian and ate mostly salads. That sounded good to me. I told my mom I wanted to become a vegetarian. When I first started, she thought it was a good idea, because it was so healthy, but recently, she's become a little worried because I basically only eat salad, and not very much of it. She hasn't totally freaked out yet though. My father hasn't seemed to notice how much weight I've lost, but I suspect Mom has been talking to him about it.

I had stopped dance lessons for a while because I was too embarrassed to go back after Ms. White made me feel so bad. But now it is time to go back. I know she is going to be very proud of me when she sees me.

POINTS TO PONDER

Although her dance teacher's comment was indeed harsh, it's clear in this scenario that Anne has a tendency to be extremely sensitive—a typical quality for a girl who is susceptible to developing an eating disorder. Recent research shows that low self-esteem, perfectionism, and a sensitive temperament are prevalent in girls who develop anorexia. Sadly, girls with these characteristics are not helped by successes—in other words, success does not boost their self-esteem, as it does in most people. Rather, their tendency to feel negatively about themselves seems impervious to successful experiences.

Sensitive teens are often not very revealing to parents about how they feel when their self-esteem is punctured, so parents need to be on the lookout for facial expressions and words that indicate that their teen needs to talk. Sometimes listening intently and offering reassurance is all that it takes to pull a teen out of a reaction to criticism or harsh words. Noticing the distress and having a well-timed, open conversation could block an extreme reaction, such as drastic dieting or another compulsive behavior aimed at numbing out negative feelings. Parents' words can also counter the perspective offered by a dance instructor or coach, who may be single-minded about the body shape and size needed for a sport. Children need challenges and feedback when they are learning a new skill, but they also need lots of room to make mistakes, and lots of support for their efforts. If they are particularly sensitive, they need even more reassurance and validation than usual, because they tend to be hard on themselves anyway.

Unfortunately, in our scenario, Anne's teacher was also hard on her, reinforcing Anne's sensitivity to the reactions of others. Her teacher was more focused on body type and weight than she was on dancing ability and enjoyment. She apparently believed that the best way to motivate was through criticism. She may have been unaware of how sensitive Anne was, and of the power and influence she had over Anne. She may also have been unaware of the triggers for an eating disorder.

We have stressed that a trigger is not a cause. The dance teacher did not cause Anne's eating disorder, but her criticism was an influential contributing factor for Anne, who apparently took corrective words very seriously. By the same token, if the dance teacher instead conveyed a positive attitude toward Anne's performance and body, she could have had the power to help to avert the onset of anorexia. Criticizing a girl's body is especially detrimental at puberty—the stage Anne was experiencing in this scenario. Puberty is a time when body consciousness is at an all-time high, because the body is changing so rapidly that it feels almost alien to the teen. Even for teens who are not particularly sensitive, self-consciousness is a given, and any additional focus, especially if it is critical, can seriously erode self-confidence. A fingernail on an abdomen can leave an indelible mark on a young girl's view of her body and of her identity, since the body and the identity are mistakenly perceived as one and the same at this time in her development.

When Anne's mother picked her up from the dance lesson and noticed that she was quiet, she could have pursued the conversation instead of stopping when Anne didn't explain. Also, Anne could have taken the initiative to give voice to her concerns and gained a new perspective by talking about her emotional reactions. It is quite possible that the other dance students weren't being as judgmental as she feared they were. Anne could have told her parents about the incident to get their take on it, but in this case, her silence kept her from seeing a different perspective and regaining her balance.

It is important for sensitive teens to check in with a trusted adult to see whether their troubling perceptions are on target. Anne's parents had already shared with her that she had a sensitive nature. They had recommended that she should try not to worry so much about what other people are thinking about her, because those people are usually just doing their own thing. A conversation started either by Anne or by her parents could have put this troubling situation in better perspective for Anne and could have prevented the impulsive reaction that led to her eating disorder.

It is important for adults to accept responsibility for their influence and their power to build up the self-esteem of children or to tear it down. Unwitting remarks from adults in positions of authority, born of their own need for the children under their instruction to excel by *their* standards, can be damaging. Even with caring comments, there may be occasions when a teen's self-esteem remains low, despite an adult's best efforts and noble intentions. However, adults should do their best to eliminate the possibility that their words are contributing to the problem instead of helping teens to feel better about themselves. Good intentions have a positive influence only if they are communicated to teens in a manner experienced as affirming, and in a way that allows for them to make mistakes and grow from their experiences.

CHANGING THE PATTERN

PARENTS

∼ Affirm your teen's appearance on a regular basis. Puberty is a time when young girls especially need affirmation, not criticism. This is even more true if the teen has an innate tendency toward low self-esteem and sensitivity.

∼ Remember that you may not be able to "fix" an overly sensitive personality, but you can help that person manage her extreme and uncomfortable reactions to criticism.

∼ Be patient with yourself, even if your best efforts to build your teen's self-esteem seem to make little difference. Keep affirming, and keep listening.

∼ If you have a sensitive teen, try to make an extra effort to meet and get to know the adults they are interacting with. Check to see if those adults understand the importance of affirmation during this critical time.

❧ Talk to teens—especially teen girls—about how their bodies will change. Explain how girls often gain weight just before puberty to prepare for childbearing but settle into a slimmer shape after the transition. This explanation can be comforting to a girl who is self-conscious and mistakenly thinks she is just becoming fat.

TEENS

❧ If you know that you are sensitive, understand that it is a gift. Sensitive people make the world a better place, because they notice and understand things that others miss. Because of your sensitivity, you will probably reach out to others in a caring way.

❧ If you tend to worry a lot, try checking in with a trusted friend or adult to see whether they think your concerns are reasonable. It's always good to get a second opinion!

❧ If your feelings have been hurt, find someone that you trust to share your hurt feelings with. Don't suffer alone when a conversation could help you to feel better.

❧ Try to focus on enjoying yourself and having fun, even when you are learning something new. Don't worry about what anybody else thinks as you learn. Everyone is attracted by that kind of carefree attitude.

❧   Remember that your body is going through rapid changes
right now. It will eventually find its rightful shape. Be
patient and give it a chance.

Scenario 10

A FINAL FAREWELL

WHEN A PARENT IS TERMINALLY ILL

Those who learned to know death, rather than to fear and fight it, become our teachers about life.
—Dr. Elisabeth Kübler-Ross

The terminal illness of a parent is very traumatic for a teen. Not only is it devastating to realize that a parent is actually going to die, but it is also incredibly sad and upsetting to live in the same house with a dying parent, who isn't acting like his usual self and needs a lot of extra attention.

Teens already worry about what friends and teachers think about everything they do, and having a parent with a terminal illness can bring up feelings of being different and cut off from normal activities. There is so much to handle at the same time: anger, sadness, and confusion about the meaning of life and death. The hardest emotion may be guilt about sometimes wishing the parent would die to end the suffering and the stress. All of these feelings are normal, but often, the teen can't bring herself to share the pain with anyone. She may try to hide the situation and deny that it is happening at all. Preoccupied with grief and guilt, and not wanting to burden the other parent, who is also overwhelmed, she can turn to an eating disorder to offer the comfort that food symbolizes, to numb out her feelings, and to give her a sense of control in at least one area of her life. Often done in secret, the eating-disordered behaviors can seem like a temporary refuge from the demands of the sick parent and the chores that the caretaking parent may ask her to do. Bingeing and purging can start as an occasional behavior and then can become an entrenched, dysfunctional coping mechanism that continues after the parent dies. While the other parent's attention is on the ill spouse, the teen can feel cut off from support and not know where else to turn for comfort.

In the following scenario, seventeen-year-old Abby is unsuccessful at reconciling all of the feelings she has about her father's illness and turns to an eating disorder when her attempts to cope do not work.

THE BELL RANG, AND I IMMEDIATELY FELT

the dread in my belly like a lead weight. I knew I had to go right home, but I couldn't seem to get up from my desk. I just sat there, watching my classmates with envy as they grabbed their backpacks and books and rushed out the door. They were happy to be free now—free to hang out with their friends, or to go play sports, or just to go home and veg out.

I used to have good excuses not to go home—track practice, tutoring freshmen, needing to go to the library. But after Dad's health took a turn for the worst last month, I had to quit track. Mom felt so bad about asking me to quit, and she explained with tears in her eyes that she just really needs my help at home. So of course I did what she asked. I've always been a good daughter.

Besides, she really does need my help. She looks so exhausted these days, even though we have a hospice nurse helping us three times a week. It's just that taking care of Dad has become pretty much a twenty-four-hour job. Because of the morphine, he sleeps on and off all day and doesn't really have a sense of time anymore. When Mom does sleep, it's on the fold-out in the living room, which I'm sure isn't very comfortable. But after we decided to bring Dad home from the hospital, their bedroom was basically turned into a hospital room, complete with a hospital bed, IVs, bedpans, and dinner trays. It would be impossible for her to get any good rest in there.

It's really hard. Our lives have been turned upside down. But it was either this, or keeping him in the hospital and going to visit him every day. The thought of Dad being alone so much was unbearable, both to me and to Mom. And even though communicating with him is pretty much impossible these days, we knew he would want to be home rather than being alone in the hospital.

"Abby? Are you okay?"

I looked up and saw Mrs. Wood standing over me. All the kids were gone already. I guess I zoned out for a while. I'm pretty exhausted myself these days.

"Oh. Yeah. I'm okay," I said, gathering my stuff and getting up. "I just spaced out."

"You seem to be spacing out a lot lately. Is everything okay? Is your father okay?"

Ugh! I hated having to talk about it. It made me so mad that Mom told the school the truth about why I had to miss so much school last month. Why didn't she just make something up, like a family reunion, or a great aunt's funeral, or a really bad case of the flu? But no. She told the principal that my dad has cancer and probably only has a few more months to live. So now, on top of all the other stress, I have to deal with pitying glances from my teachers and weird looks from my friends. I don't know how they found out, but they must know. The way they shy away from me, you'd think it was *me* who had cancer, and that it was contagious. Luckily, I have a couple of good friends who really care about me. I can talk to them, but I know they don't know what to say sometimes. Plus, I never have time to hang out with them anymore, and they certainly don't want to come over to my house. And I don't blame them. It's so depressing there.

"No, my dad isn't really okay, Mrs. Wood. He's dying." I know I sounded snotty, but I didn't know how else to answer the question. "Thanks for your concern, though," I said, trying to sound sincere.

Mrs. Wood put her hand on my shoulder. "Abby," she said. "I know how hard this is for you and your mom. I think you could use some extra help. Have you thought about visiting Mr. Paulsen? He's really good." Mr. Paulsen was our school counselor.

"Not really," I answered. "I'll think about it, though," I added, even though I didn't really mean it. I just wanted to get out of there as quickly as possible.

"Do think about it, Abby. If you want, I can call your mom to talk with her about it. I really think you need some extra support right now," she said.

"Please don't call my mom, Mrs. Wood. I appreciate your concern, and I'll think about talking to Mr. Paulsen, but please don't call my mom. She has enough on her mind right now."

Mrs. Wood nodded and watched me leave. It was so good to be out in the fresh air, out of that room, which suddenly had become so stifling. But once I started on my path home, I felt my pace slow down again. I knew how it would be the minute I walked in the door. Mom would be pacing in the kitchen, on the phone with a doctor or my aunt, and the TV in the living room would be on. She likes to keep the TV on at all hours now, even when she's sleeping. She says the talking in the background comforts her. It probably also helps drown out at least a few of Dad's groans and calls to her. That might sound harsh, but it's not. I understand. Because of the morphine, he's kind of in a dream state most of the time, so sometimes he just calls out for me or Mom but doesn't actually need or want anything. It's like he's talking in his sleep, but his eyes are open.

When I got home, there would be dishes in the sink and dirty sheets to be washed. I'd need to go upstairs and open the bedroom windows because Mom always forgets to let some fresh air in. Mom would wave to me from the phone and look at me sympathetically. When she got off the phone, she'd find me and ask me how my day was. I'd be able to see in her eyes how sorry she was that I never get to relax and have fun anymore. But I guess we both know things won't be like this forever. The way Dad's health is going, he will probably be gone before the end of the fall term.

It makes me feel horrible, absolutely horrible to admit it, but part of me can't wait until all this is over. But then, when I think about what it will be like this Christmas—when it's just me and Mom, without Dad to videotape every single second of the holiday while telling dorky jokes—I get so sad I can't stand it. I don't understand how I can feel both ways inside, and it's tearing me apart.

On the way home, I stopped at the convenience store again. Mom's been giving me $20 a week lately. I don't know if it's guilt or what. She just said that I've been helping her so much, it's the least she could do. So once or twice a week I stop at the store and buy a huge bag of chips, candy, cupcakes, donuts, whatever I feel like. On those days, I go through the side gate when I get home. I sit in the backyard, under a tree, where Mom can't see me, and I stuff myself with everything I bought. When I'm eating, I just zone out completely, and before I know it, everything I bought is gone.

And then the panic sets in. I look down and see my belly pooching out, and I feel disgusting. So I get up to take care of the mess I've made of myself. I go in through the back door. For some reason, Mom never asks me why I don't go in through the front. She hasn't noticed how much weight I've lost, either. She probably just thinks it's because we don't get much time to have regular meals these days. When I come in, she just waves to me from the kitchen phone. I go into my room, dump my stuff, and head straight for the bathroom to get rid of all the junk I just ate. I lock the door behind me, but I never have to worry about Mom hearing what I'm doing in there, what with the TV going all the time. When I'm finished, I feel clean and pure again. I wash my face and brush my teeth. I take a deep breath, and then I feel strong enough to go to the bedroom to see Dad.

POINTS TO PONDER

Abby obviously had many conflicting emotions waging war within her. She had a strong sense of loyalty to her family and wanted to be there for her mother, who was obviously overloaded with caretaking. She also felt angry about her situation and knew she was missing out on a lot of fun with her friends. In addition, she felt embarrassed about the fact that her teachers—and possibly, her classmates—knew what was happening. She was sad about losing her father, but she also felt terribly guilty for the sense of relief she knew she'd feel when he was gone.

Her anger and guilt were probably mounting, but she didn't know what to do with those feelings. Because she apparently was such a "good" child, we might be able to guess that anger was not acceptable to her or to her family. Still, her anger slipped out in tiny ways, such as when Mrs. Wood asked her about her father after school.

Abby's emotional confusion was fertile ground for the onset of an eating disorder and also made it difficult for her to reach out for help. Even though her eating disorder was only about a month old, we know she had reached the second stage of bulimia: using the bingeing and purging to numb emotions. If she were characteristic of most teens with bulimia, she would have gone through an initial stage in which she used the behavior only to lose weight. In this first stage, a person usually believes she can stop at any time. As the behavior increases, she transitions into a second stage: getting hooked on the numbing nature of the binge-purge ritual and turning to this source of comfort when she is upset.

If Abby is not helped, she could move into a third stage: bingeing and purging as part of a pervasive lifestyle that is as persistent and habitual as brushing one's teeth. If she reaches this stage, recovery will be much more difficult.

To add to the challenge of Abby's emotional confusion, her mom was so preoccupied with her father's medical crisis that she was unable to give her daughter the attention she needed so much. While her mother was not responsible for Abby's problem or for her recovery, her perceptive attention to Abby's need may have brought about the opening that Abby needed to talk about how she was feeling. If her mother noticed or realized that Abby had unspoken feelings about her father's illness, she could have started a conversation that would have made it easier for Abby to admit her struggle with overeating. This degree of intimacy could have increased the chance that Abby would be open to entering a solid recovery process.

It could be that Abby's mom suspected that something was wrong, but that the thought of Abby having an eating disorder would be far too much for her to take on top of her husband's illness. Considering the circumstances, it's entirely plausible that her mom was just completely unaware of Abby's eating disorder. It may have been that Abby needed to take the first step in this case to start a conversation, unless her mother could widen her focus long enough to pick up on the signs. She might have had the presence of mind to ask Abby why she came through the back door sometimes. She might have realized that the TV needed to be turned off once in a while to create a sense of peace, and after doing so, she might have heard Abby vomiting in the bathroom. But she was just trying to survive emotionally and didn't notice what Abby was doing.

Knowing that you are going to lose a parent while still being a teenager can be scary and devastating. Adolescence is often a time of many doubts about oneself and decisions about the future, and to feel abandoned at this time can add grief that derails the normal progression of a teen's development. It is also a time when family communication is essential but often difficult. It is hard to share feelings that hurt and are hard to describe. But a little goes a long way. If you feel overwhelmed, start small. A tiny opening into the heart can naturally widen with time and patience, and trust. It doesn't matter who breaks the ice and starts the conversation, or dares to cry. It just matters that someone does.

By making sure to create the time and environment for regular communication about the difficult thoughts and emotions that come with an experience like this, teens and parents can show one another the love and support that each person needs. The comfort that comes from having an honest emotional conversation not only fortifies a teen against the false sense of comfort that an eating disorder seems to promise—it also deepens her relationship to her surviving parent, as well as her relationship to herself.

CHANGING THE PATTERN

PARENTS

❧ If your spouse is terminally ill and you have a teen who is grieving with you, talk about your real feelings with your teen. Pretending the problem doesn't exist can build a wall between you.

❧ Think about how hard it would be to have a parent dying if you were still a teen. The suffering is different from yours as a spouse, but just as difficult.

❧ If you are overwhelmed, give yourself permission to get help from friends, a support group, or a therapist. When you are supported, it will be easier to reach out to your teen.

❧ Observe how your teen is handling the problem, and if you see unusual and worrisome behaviors, tell her your concerns and get her the help she needs.

TEENS

❧ Find someone to talk to about your parent's illness or seek counseling. The fears, frustrations, and sadness are natural and need to be expressed.

❧ Try journaling, listening to music, taking a bubble bath. Take care of yourself to balance out the pain.

❧ Tell your ill parent what he or she means to you. Later, you won't have regrets about not expressing your love and appreciation.

❧ Open up a conversation with your well parent about your feelings. Your parent may need the closeness as much as you do.

⬡   Remember: An eating disorder will never numb you enough to make the pain go away for good. It is not the answer to your grief and will only make your problems worse.

SUPPLEMENTARY READING

FOR TEENS

The Grieving Teen: A Guide for Teenagers and Their Friends, by Helen Fitzgerald

Straight Talk about Death for Teenagers: How to Cope with Losing Someone You Love, by Earl A. Grollman

Scenario 11

WHO'S THE FAVORITE?

WHEN SIBLING RIVALRY
CREATES BARRIERS

Siblings are the people we practice on, the people who teach us about fairness and cooperation and kindness and caring— quite often the hard way.

—Pamela Dugdale

All children tend to compare themselves with their siblings, wondering how their parents see them in relationship to one another. It's a natural and common tendency, and it can help them learn valuable life lessons about how to cooperate with others, fight fair, and deal with conflicting feelings about another person. However, it can also create doubts about who is "the best," how to be unique, and how to maintain self-esteem if they seem to come in second. When parents compare their children to one another, they can reinforce a negative process of self-evaluation, even when they are trying to highlight their children's individual differences in an effort to improve self-esteem.

In the following scenario, fourteen-year-old Jenny struggles to create her own niche—a way to stand out—in the face of her brother's teasing and her sister's apparent perfection.

IT WAS MY FIRST DAY OF HIGH SCHOOL, AND

everyone was staring at me in amazement and admiration. Some of my friends didn't even recognize me! On some of their faces, I could see jealousy. But I didn't care. *It serves them right for parading their skinny little bodies around the school last year and teasing me about my hips and thighs,* I thought. *Now it's my turn!*

Walking down the hallways on the way to my classes, I felt victorious. What an accomplishment, to have lost fifty pounds over the summer! I felt better than I have ever felt in my life—even better than the day I won first place in the "Little Miss Princess" contest, the most prestigious beauty contest I ever won. I was only five years old then, but I still remember how incredible it was to walk down the ramp with the gold crown on my blond curls, carrying a bundle of red roses. My sister, Alicia, and I used to win contest after contest in those days; sometimes Alicia would win, and sometimes I won. We were both pretty, and we loved the attention, especially from our parents. As we got older, though, we started getting really competitive. Even though Mom and Dad loved the attention we got for our contests, they made us stop entering because of our fights. I was relieved in some ways, because I was always worrying about not winning, but I also missed the smiles on my parents' faces when I was crowned.

I was mad at all those girls who teased me last year. I could hear them calling me "pudgy" behind my back and saying that they didn't want to hang out with me because I was getting fat. I was even more mad at my little brother, Jed. His comments had been stinging me for years. He always knew exactly what to say about my weight when he wanted to make me feel bad about myself. Just because he is such a soccer star doesn't give him the right to be a jerk.

My parents always said I wasn't overweight, but I knew they were just trying to make me feel better about myself. They said my brother was just being mean and knew that a comment about my weight would upset me more than anything. They were right! I hated him for saying I was fat. My brother didn't know it, but sometimes I disappeared into my room and just cried for hours because of his awful comments.

It didn't help that Alicia was perfect: smart, beautiful, and a goody-two-shoes around Mom and Dad. Worst of all, she was homecoming queen her sophomore year! How was I supposed to stand out in high school with that kind of competition? It wasn't fair. I won contests just as often as she did when we were little, but then I started to feel fat and ugly.

Nobody really tried to make me feel better about any of that stuff. Of course, I wasn't telling my parents how bad I really felt. If they knew, they might have helped.

But that is all behind me now. I will never feel that way again. Now I am skinnier than Alicia by far. It feels great to be the only skinny one. It was so worth it to deprive myself of pizza, ice cream, pasta, and potatoes! At first it was hard, and on many nights I would go to bed with my stomach growling, but now I don't miss food at all. The hungrier I feel, the more powerful I feel.

Last week, at my physical, the doctor expressed concern about my rapid weight loss, but I didn't care. *What does he know about what is important to me?* I thought. No one can pop my bubble now, not even a stupid doctor. My mother told the doctor I was just going through a phase and would soon stop this silly weight-loss thing. If you want to know my opinion, I think she was secretly happy that I had lost weight. But who knows? Dad didn't say much when Mom told him what the doctor said. He just turned to me and told me to eat more at meals. He said he would remind me so the doctor would stop worrying. I think they didn't want the doctor to think they were bad parents. Anyway, I wasn't worried. I knew what I wanted and how I was going to get there. It would be easy enough to keep my dad off my back. He wasn't home much at dinner and wouldn't notice if I lost more weight. If Mom was secretly happy about how I looked, she wouldn't say anything either.

Finally, I have a niche that is all my own. I have found my *own* way to be special, different from my brother and sister, different from anything any of my friends can ever achieve. Maybe Mom and even Dad will finally see that my sister is not the only one in this family who deserves recognition.

After feeling today's triumphant success, I made a silent resolution: *Never again* will I weigh more than a hundred pounds. Maybe I'll even shoot for ninety. The thinner, the better. And I will make sure that no one ever discovers my secret—my own special solution, reserved for times when I slip up and eat something on the forbidden-food list. Sweets and chips are the foods that usually worry me and send me to the store to buy laxatives to undo the damage. After all, it's normal to eat sweets sometimes. My mom doesn't know that I am using my allowance and my babysitting money to buy laxatives. Sometimes they give me stomach cramps, but it's worth it. As long as I am skinny, I can endure a little pain. After all, it's going really well. Alicia and Jed will never be as thin as I am.

POINTS TO PONDER

In order to follow the development of Jenny's eating disorder, we need to look at her history. When she was five years old, she was in a beauty contest, which may have contributed to having good feelings about herself based on her appearance. Being in additional beauty contests created a belief in the importance of looking and acting perfect. This belief may have been reinforced when she saw how happy her parents were when she won. We see that she also loved being in the limelight and the thrill of being announced a winner.

Her parents' intention with the beauty contests may have been simply to help Jenny to be more poised and to feel good about herself. On the other hand, they may have enjoyed the personal recognition that their daughters' success brought them. Parents who have work to do on their own self-esteem may attempt to gain positive feelings about themselves through their children's accomplishments. Although children may enjoy winning trophies, they don't benefit from being seen by family members as trophies. Regardless of their intentions with the beauty contests, Jenny's parents needed to be sure to shift their focus when she became a teen and convey to her that she is loved for deeper aspects of her personality, instead of for her accomplishments, looks, and body type.

Certainly the beauty pageants did not cause the eating disorder, but the family focus on them may indicate not only their need to shine through their children, but also a tendency to compare one child to another and to motivate each child through competition. This can develop into an unhealthy form of sibling rivalry.

It was obvious that Jenny did not feel she had her own unique niche, different from her brother's and her sister's. This may be more common among middle children, who don't have the privileges of the oldest or get the attention they feel is granted to the youngest. Jenny was searching desperately for her place in the family structure. If, for example, one sibling is smart and another is athletic, the "most attractive" or "thinnest" niche may seem to be the only one available. Unfortunately, many parents with good intentions reinforce this kind of thinking. In an attempt to help their children see themselves as unique individuals, parents will often describe their children in this way: "Bobbie is my smart one, Linda is my athlete, and Jenny is my pretty one." Instead of reacting to their parents' attempt with a renewed sense of being unique, a child may sense that only one child can have a particular strength—and once that niche is taken, they have to find another way to excel or be loved.

In Jenny's case, this niche became achieving an unnatural thinness and led to her eating disorder. Laxative abuse is a purging technique that is particularly dangerous because it can cause dehydration and potassium depletion, both of which can lead to cardiac problems. In addition, laxatives are habit-forming and cause abdominal cramping. Unfortunately, bulimia nervosa became Jenny's misguided way to create a new identity among her siblings, and her parents were unaware of her dangerous habit. They also seemed to be only partially aware of the seriousness of her condition.

There are times when parents seem to do everything within their power to foster a sense of self-worth in their children, and still, a given child may strive for perfect grades or every award at school. Although we don't understand completely how individual temperament affects children, we know that children can put their own spin on their parents' words and drive themselves, regardless of how hard their parents try to take off the pressure. Parents do well not to blame themselves, but instead to examine their own style of parenting and take into consideration their child's unique sensitivities and insecurities.

Everyone wants to find a niche and be valued for being unique, but there are usually shared interests among children, and so it often happens that two children can become competitive in a certain activity or way. Parents need to remember to give each of their children feedback that is meant for them alone, not in the context of a sibling's performance or characteristics. This is especially true with teens, who are forging their own identities and can become confused by well-intended but harmful comparisons made to siblings.

The best attitude parents can have is to see each of their children as unique individuals who have their own personalities, strengths, tendencies, and interests. Sometimes those unique qualities overlap with their siblings' characteristics, and sometimes they don't. Parents need to be enough in tune with their teens' needs and goals to notice when rivalry with siblings is causing pursuit of a niche that may be harmful or unnatural. Handling sibling rivalry is a challenge, but with good communication and careful attention, families can steer clear of the damaging aspects of this kind of competition.

CHANGING THE PATTERN

PARENTS

∼ Remember that your child is a unique human being, not necessarily a reflection of yourself. Check in with yourself to make sure you do not see your children as a vehicle for boosting your own self-esteem.

∼ Comment on your children's inner strengths on a regular basis. Don't forget the less obvious ones, such as setting the table well, or having a nice smile.

∼ Avoid comparing your children to one another or labeling them. This can only foster resentment between siblings or contribute to feelings of inferiority or superiority.

∼ Let your children know that you love them unconditionally and simply because they are your children—not because of their accomplishments.

TEENS

∼ Remember: If you have a sister or brother who excels at a certain thing, that doesn't mean you can't excel at it too!

∼ Strive to be the best *you* can be. Trying to be like someone else will just make you unhappy.

∽   If you get teased by a sibling so much that it affects how
you feel about yourself, tell him or her that it bothers you.
Ask your parents for support.

∽   If you find yourself seeking a niche that involves
purging behavior like laxative abuse, admit to yourself
how dangerous it is and tell your parents. It is better to
get help than to suffer in silence and develop a serious
medical problem.

∽   Love your brothers and sisters for who they are, and
try not to compare yourself to them. Each one of you is
wonderfully unique.

Scenario 12

IN CONTROL

WHEN TEENS SHOW SIGNS OF
PERFECTIONISM OR OCD

*Perfectionism is the voice of the oppressor, the enemy of the
people. It will keep you cramped and insane your whole life.*
—Anne Lamott

In this achievement-oriented society, many teens try to be as
perfect as possible in multiple areas. The goal might be perfect
grades, perfect popularity, or perfect athletic skills—or all of
the above. When extreme, this pursuit of perfectionism can be
defined as obsessive-compulsive disorder (OCD). A teen who is
in the grips of this disorder struggles with obsessive thoughts,
and develops compulsive behaviors to gain relief from the
obsessive thoughts.

When body shape and size become an additional target for
perfectionism, a serious eating disorder can result. Trying to be as

thin as possible can lead to a dangerously low weight that never seems low enough. A sense of failure sets in, and self-esteem can be seriously compromised. When teens suffer from the combination of OCD and an eating disorder, parents can be baffled by how to advise them and offer support. In the following scenario, fifteen-year-old Sarah is in the grips of OCD, which leads to eating behaviors that cross the line into anorexia nervosa.

THE FOOD RITUALS BEGAN ONE YEAR AGO

when I started high school. I have a certain way I like to have my food arranged on my plate and a certain order in which I can eat things. Vegetables always get eaten first, then meat, and then potatoes. The order can never vary. During the day, I hate having to eat at the school cafeteria. The food is so greasy and disgusting. Sometimes I take my lunch, but sometimes I just give it away or eat an apple. Mom doesn't know I don't eat my lunch. Surprisingly, she isn't even suspicious about the fact that I've lost fifteen pounds in the last two months. My periods seem to have stopped too, but I haven't told Mom yet. I heard that's a sure sign of anorexia, and the last thing I want in the world is for Mom and Dad to be disappointed in me. "Anorexia" would be a scary word to them, and they would jump all over me. I have to find out how to have a perfect body without worrying them. That won't be easy, but I'll find a way.

I can't remember exactly when I began counting stairs and not stepping on cracks in the sidewalk. It might have been in fourth or fifth grade. But I do remember that I was twelve when I had to start arranging my stuffed animals on the shelf and on my bed in a certain order, or else I couldn't go to sleep at night. I also *have* to have my socks and underwear arranged in my drawers by color, and because doing that takes up so much room, Mom had to buy me a new dresser.

It doesn't seem like my friends have to have things a certain way all the time. It's kind of embarrassing when they come over to spend the night, and they see how I'm always arranging things a certain way. But I can't help it! I feel like if I don't do things that way, something horrible will happen to me, or to my sister, or to Mom or Dad. But if I do follow the rules, everything will be fine.

I'm the same way in all aspects of my life. I'm a straight-A student, and I play first-chair flute in the school orchestra, and I'm class secretary. I'm on my way to having a model-perfect body too. If I can just lose fifteen more pounds, I'll be down to ninety, and then I'll know I've reached perfection. Everything in my life up to now has shown me: I can accomplish anything I want if I make up my mind to go for it.

My parents love me very much. They tell me I am wonderful just the way I am. As long as my grades are good and I don't get in trouble, they are fine with what I do. I hope they keep focusing on all my great achievements in school so that they don't start noticing that I am losing a bunch of weight. I can't let them try to stop me from getting the perfect body! It's the only goal I haven't achieved yet.

POINTS TO PONDER

Sarah represents a subtype of anorexic who suffers from obsessive-compulsive disorder as well as from an eating disorder. Obsessive-compulsive disorder (OCD) is a mental disorder characterized by worrisome, repetitive thoughts followed by ritualistic habits and behaviors designed to "magically" wipe out the obsessive thoughts.

Sarah had recurrent thoughts because she feared being imperfect. These thoughts were followed by repetitive behaviors, such as counting and arranging her stuffed animals in a certain order—unconsciously designed to reassure herself that her worst fears would not materialize. OCD seems to be linked to an inherited predisposition to anxiety, as well as to environmental factors, such as societal pressure and pressure by family members to meet their standards of perfection. Some families emphasize athletics, some emphasize academics, and some focus on physical beauty. Many parents focus on perfection in *every* area, which certainly ups the ante. In Sarah's situation, her parents wanted her to have good grades and may or may not have been pressuring her in other ways. Sarah seemed to be pressuring *herself* to be perfect, and her parents may have been wringing their hands, not knowing how to stop her.

Unfortunately, the pressure to be perfect often becomes more pronounced when a young boy or girl reaches puberty—a time of added stress because of the new challenges that come with being a teenager. When Sarah reached high school, she was faced with new concerns, such as competing academically, dealing with a changing body, thinking about her future after high school, and becoming more independent from her parents. In addition, she was probably bombarded with society's obsession with thinness. Since she already had a tendency to focus on being perfect, she was much more susceptible to becoming obsessive and compulsive about her weight, her body shape, and her eating habits. Her weight may have seemed "controllable," and this pursuit of thinness may have helped her to shift the focus away from areas of her life that seemed scary and harder to manage, such as being attractive to guys, getting good grades, or accepting her adult body.

What can parents, teachers, coaches, and other professionals do to help teens like Sarah relax their rules and rituals? The answer is not simple, and is usually reached by trial and error. First of all, because of the probable genetic component, a psychiatrist or family doctor can often help by prescribing medications that address OCD as well as the eating disorder. In addition, parents can begin to send the message to their children that they are loved simply for "being" and not just for what they can accomplish.

Teens like Sarah have a much better chance of escaping a full-blown eating disorder if their parents and other concerned adults recognize the early signs of excessive perfectionism. These adults can then begin to offer emotional support for an adolescent's concerns about her changing body, her fear of not succeeding academically, or her desire to be popular. If this support is not enough, they can seek professional help.

Parents often have to examine first their own tendencies to strive for perfection, or to feel good about themselves only when their children are outstanding in athletics or academics. If a mother, for example, is suffering from the Superwoman complex herself—thinking she has to be a perfect wife, mother, career woman, and beauty queen—this message will surely get conveyed to her daughter. Teachers and coaches are also an important influence, because they are in the business of encouraging outstanding performance on the part of students. Doing one's best should be encouraged; perfection at the risk of one's physical or mental health is excessive pressure.

Even in the absence of family pressure, some kids are born with OCD tendencies and need extra help with their perfectionism. When teens bring this temperament into the world, it may be more advantageous for parents and other concerned adults to help them *manage* it than to try to convince them to *change* something that feels to them like a part of their personality. Management skills are especially important during puberty, when added stress often increases the anxiety and makes the symptoms worse.

With the help of effective therapy and strong parental understanding and support, perfectionism and OCD do not have to be crippling. A more relaxed approach to life and activities— one that emphasizes enjoyment instead of perfect performance— can replace obsessive thoughts and compulsive rituals. Eating disorders lose their hold when you focus on being who you truly are, each moment, instead of worrying about all of the ways you are falling short. Recovery begins the moment you decide that you are wonderful, just the way you are.

CHANGING THE PATTERN

PARENTS

❧ Pay attention to signs of obsessive thoughts or compulsive behaviors that may accompany symptoms of an eating disorder.

❧ Recognize that eating disorders and obsessive-compulsive disorder are not only emotional disorders but also medical conditions that need attention. Help is available for both conditions through psychotherapists, medical doctors, and dietitians. Sometimes medication is an important part of this treatment regimen.

❧ Encourage teens to do their best instead of giving subtle or direct messages that only perfect performance, perfect behavior, or a perfect body are acceptable.

TEENS

❧ Perfection is an impossible goal. Doing your personal best is much more important.

∾   If you are focused on being perfect, you may miss other parts of your life that will actually bring more joy—such as enjoying being with friends, enjoying nature, and engaging in sports and music for the pure joy of being in the moment.

∾   If you feel anxious, have thoughts that run through your head and won't stop, need things to be a certain way, or need a certain routine to feel "okay," let your parents or an adult you trust know what you are going through. They can help.

SUPPLEMENTARY READING:

FOR PARENTS AND TEENS

Freeing our Families from Perfectionism, by Thomas S. Greenspon

Never Good Enough: How to Use Perfectionism to Your Advantage Without Letting It Ruin Your Life, by Monica Ramirez Basco

Perfectionism: What's Bad about Being Too Good, by M. Adderholdt and Jan Goldberg

Rewind, Replay, Repeat, by Jeff Bell

When Perfect Isn't Good Enough: Strategies for Coping with Perfectionism, by Marten M. Antony and Richard Swinson

Scenario 13

WHATEVER IT TAKES TO WIN

WHEN ATHLETES FEEL COMPELLED
TO CONTROL THEIR WEIGHT

Any movement toward self-improvement must be propelled
not by disgust and self-rejection, but by a realistic acceptance
of who we already are and a desire to be the best possible
version of that reality.

—Marcia Germaine Hutchinson

In some sports—such as gymnastics, dancing, wrestling, track, cross-country running, and ice skating—young athletes are often pressured to maintain a low body weight and low body-fat levels. Unfortunately, because most kids think being as skinny as possible will help them excel at their sport, they will often experiment with extreme weight-loss practices. But the fact is that being undernourished while trying to compete can actually hurt performance. Nutrition deprivation and dehydration can also have serious health consequences, because active, growing adolescents need even more nutrients and calories than usual to ensure proper growth and development.

In the following scenario, fifteen-year-old Scott wants desperately to wrestle in the lower weight category, where he has achieved previous success in middle school. He believes that if he can stay in the same category, he will have a better chance to prove himself to his new high school coach, and his dad.

———————————

I WAS REALLY LOOKING FORWARD TO BEING

on my high school wrestling team. At Andrade Middle School, I was a pretty good wrestler—everyone thought so—and I couldn't wait to show my new coach what I could do. I'd always been a skinny guy, so wrestling in the lower weights was never a problem before. But over the summer, I'd grown about four inches and gained twenty pounds!

Plus, my appetite is huge all the time. I'm always hungry! It made me feel really uneasy as the date of the tryouts approached. I knew I'd have to step on the scale, and I was really scared about what the consequences would be.

The day came to weigh in, and as we entered the gym, the coach greeted us all with a hearty handshake and instructed us to have a seat on the bleachers. After we were all seated, the coach welcomed us and introduced the trainer, who explained his role in working with the team. His job was to help each of us achieve our best.

It turns out, I was right to be scared. When I got on the scale, the trainer confirmed my worst fears. I was over the weight limit for wrestling in the lower weights, meaning I would have to compete against kids much bigger than me. I'd never win a match! The trainer pulled me aside at the end of tryouts and said he would be happy to work with me so I would be more comfortable wrestling in the higher weight class. No way was I going to do that! I knew I'd get my butt kicked and disappoint everyone who was counting on me.

I went home determined to lose some pounds so that the next time I weighed in, I would make weight. No way was I going to go up against those big guys and look like a fool. My parents were so proud of my record in middle school, and I didn't want to disappoint them—especially Dad, who'd been a high school wrestler himself. I skipped dinner that night, telling Mom I didn't feel good. When I woke up the next day, I was starving, but I only allowed myself an apple as I ran out the door to catch the bus. I ate a big salad at lunch, and it felt good just to chew on something. It was really hard to pass up all the rest of the food in the cafeteria line. Everything looked *so good*—things I'd never even consider eating before seemed to be calling my name. Not only was I starving, but I was really thirsty too, since I wasn't allowing myself to drink very much either. Restricting fluids was another quick weight-loss trick I'd heard some of the guys on my team talking about.

Five days went by, and I was pleased with myself. I'd dropped five pounds! My coach congratulated me on my success. The trainer gave me the evil eye, but I didn't care. I'd done what I had to do. Although I felt physically awful, I was encouraged. I just wished I didn't feel so angry and depressed all the time. I knew I should be eating more, but losing weight was the most important thing in my life right now. It took every bit of energy I had to not chow down at lunch and load up my tray with all the food I could get my hands on, instead of just buying the salad I made myself eat. I was so hungry I could eat a horse.

Being with my friends—even being with my girlfriend—didn't seem to matter. It was easier not be around other people right now. I didn't need them making comments about what I was or wasn't eating. Besides, I wasn't in the mood to be social. When I walked my girlfriend to class this morning, she asked, "Is there anything wrong? You haven't been much fun to be around these past few days. You seem so preoccupied. Are you angry at me? Please talk to me."

I mumbled something and walked away, wondering, *What is wrong with me? I can always talk to Katie.* Oh, whatever, I'll have to figure that stuff out later. Right now I just have to stay focused and lose this weight. Even if I have to diet for the entire season so I can wrestle in the lower weights—I'll do what I have to do. I can't disappoint my dad.

POINTS TO PONDER

In this scenario, Scott was willing to starve himself to make weight rather than risk disappointing himself, his coach, and his dad with the poor performance he expected, had he been forced to wrestle boys bigger than him. Striving for a sense of control over a body that seemed to be growing out of control, he was on his way to developing an eating disorder. Whether the pressure from his dad and coach was real or imagined, Scott might not have jeopardized his health like this if communication had been more open, and if everyone involved had been supplied with proper education, understanding, and support.

In addition to starving himself, Scott resorted to reducing his liquid intake. Competition or training while dehydrated is extremely dangerous, because it prevents sweating and decreases the ability of an athlete to regulate his body temperature. Fluid losses and resulting electrolyte disturbances can increase the risk of cardiac arrhythmias, renal damage, impaired performance, and injury. Restricting both calories and fluid can affect metabolism, body composition (the ratio of fat to muscle), and overall health. In addition to those dangers, Scott's growth and development may have been affected adversely if this kind of behavior were occurring during a time when he was growing rapidly.

The high-schooler is not only growing physically, but is also growing academically, socially, and psychologically. Severe dieting affects both the mind and body. As illustrated above, Scott experienced moodiness, poor concentration, poor decision-making, and social withdrawal. Athletes who have a drive for thinness to achieve a perceived goal, at any cost, are at risk for developing an eating disorder.

It is unlikely that Scott realized what his decision to starve himself could result in: damaged health, poor performance, and problems in relationships. He also probably did not understand that his mood swings, lack of energy, and feelings of isolation were a direct result of severely restricting fluid and calorie intake.

Because body-image and eating problems are extremely difficult to change once they have been established, it is important that parents, teachers, and coaches work to prevent these problems from developing in the first place. It is also important that parents of athletes communicate with their sons and daughters—and with their coaches and teachers as well—about expectations for their involvement in sports. For many teens who participate in sports, the coach's word is truth. That's why it is very important for parents to be aware of what the coach is saying—or not saying—to their athletes about training and nutrition. It is also important to determine whether the coach's focus is on the teen's well-being or on their performance.

It is important to communicate with teens about how poor nutrition harms performance, and how proper eating can help them achieve their personal best. Had Scott taken the opportunity to listen to what the trainer had to say, he may have actually achieved more success in his high school wrestling career. Rather than being preoccupied with making weight, he could have been concentrating on learning everything he could about technique and strategy.

CHANGING THE PATTERN

PARENTS

❧ Know that males are more likely than females to diet for the purpose of improving athletic performance. Diets are dangerous and are often the precursor to an eating disorder.

❧ If your teen makes drastic changes in his routine or eating behavior, check in with him and problem-solve together.

❧ Help your teen to meet his nutritional needs by providing a variety of wholesome foods and by encouraging regular meals. He will perform better, both during his athletic events and in the classroom.

❧ Whatever the activity, encourage your young athlete to participate for the experience of being a part of something bigger than himself, and for the enjoyment of the sport. Take the focus off performance.

❧ Talk to your teen athlete about nutrition, conditioning, and weight training—and about the dangers inherent in "making weight" by starving or allowing himself to become dehydrated.

✤ Make sure your teen's coach is on the same page as you regarding these important issues.

TEENS

✤ Know that it's normal for a teenager's appetite to grow suddenly. Trust what your body needs.

✤ Know that it is counterproductive to lose weight rapidly before an event. Depleted muscle glycogen and dehydration will take their toll and can hurt rather than enhance your health and performance.

✤ Remember: If you feel thirsty, you are already dehydrated. Trying to lose weight by reducing liquid intake is dangerous.

✤ Participate in sports for the love of the game, not just to win. Sports can help you to learn self-discipline and teamwork and increase your self-esteem—all skills that will help you in the game of life.

Scenario 14

THE RUNNER'S HIGH

WHEN ATHLETIC EUPHORIA
BECOMES AN ADDICTION

In everything the middle course is best; all things in excess bring trouble.

—Plautus

Being active and exercising regularly is part of a healthy lifestyle. Unfortunately, the eating-disordered individual will often take it to extremes. Compulsive or extreme exercise is dangerous, especially for teens, whose bodies are growing and developing. The addictive nature of excessive exercise is also cause for concern, because it offers built-in reinforcement. It increases the endorphin levels, providing the individual with a sense of well-being. The compulsive exerciser will push herself to achieve this high or sense of well-being even though she may be seriously and perhaps permanently compromising her health.

In the following scenario seventeen-year-old Leslie loves to run for the pure pleasure of it, but she gradually becomes addicted to the high she feels while running. Almost without her realizing it, her morning routine begins to spiral out of control, becoming a way for her to cope with family problems.

RUNNING MEANS EVERYTHING TO ME. I NEVER consider missing my morning run, not even when I'm not feeling good. Waking up early, to the sound of birds chirping, is my favorite part of the day. While everyone else is still sleeping, I get up and get dressed as quietly as I can. Then I tiptoe down the stairs, unlatch the door, and sit down on the bench outside the door to put on my shoes. I stretch for a minute or two, start the iPod, and take off down the lane. The wind blows through my hair, and I breathe in the fresh air, relishing this time alone—time to think and be with nature. The route is so familiar I could do it blindfolded. It's very comforting, and I especially enjoy my morning runs in the winter and early spring, because it's still dark out when I leave, but the sun comes up by the time I'm done.

It wasn't like I decided to add an extra hour to my morning run. It just started happening. I never sleep very well anymore, and once, when I woke up at 4:30 A.M., I decided I might as well get up and go. After that, I realized that not only could I run for three hours straight, but also that doing so felt better than a two-hour run. But I have to be careful that no one in my family catches on that I've started working out more. Mom would have a fit if she knew I was running three hours every morning. She already doesn't like the fact that I go to the gym every afternoon to work out. "It's too much," she says. But she's wrong. How can exercise be bad for you?

When I start my morning run, I'm always a little stiff at first, but the soreness disappears once I get into a normal rhythm. Besides, when it hurts, I know I'm *really* working my body. The sensation of my feet hitting the pavement starts to become soothing and hypnotic. I feel in control again, and usually, the next time I glance down at my watch, I can be happy knowing I've already burned a hundred calories. All my stress just seems to melt away.

I've been really upset lately because things at home have been so strange. I can't quite put my finger on it, but my parents seem really tense and unhappy around each other. They try to put up a good front, but I can tell something is wrong. When I asked Mom about it, she just got annoyed and said, "Oh Leslie, don't be so dramatic! We're fine."

But it doesn't *feel* fine—especially at dinnertime, which I've started to dread. Mom and Dad just stare at their plates, avoiding eye contact and hardly saying a word. If Dad ate any faster, I think he might choke to death. My little brother, Sammy, is completely clueless, of course. He just acts like everything is normal. But it's driving me nuts!

It seems like everyone is wrapped up in their own little world. No one really notices or even seems to care when I make excuses sometimes—like having a headache or not feeling good—to avoid eating with them. I'm usually not hungry anyway, and it helps me avoid all those extra calories.

And after I added an extra hour to my run that first time, I made a discovery. I ran so hard that morning that I threw up in the park's bushes on the way home. At first I thought it was awful and felt a little dizzy, but then I realized that all that pressure that usually starts to build up in my chest on the way back home was gone. The combination of running and throwing up makes me feel almost normal, and it wipes out any guilt I might have about what I ate the day before.

Running is the only thing that makes me feel confident. I love the feeling of being totally empty and clean. Even those annoying hunger pangs have disappeared. When I get back home after my runs, I stop for an extra second or two at the hall mirror on the way to the bedroom. I look in the mirror and see how much progress I've made. I think it won't be long before I'm a size 2.

POINTS TO PONDER

In this scenario, Leslie showed a strong need to control something in her life. Her parents' relationship was faltering, and no one was willing to talk about it. This avoidance of reality can be frightening to a young person—it threatens the very foundation of the family, which is their security. Leslie couldn't control what was happening in her parents' marriage, but she could control her exercise and what she put in her mouth.

Leslie was a compulsive exerciser and, as is common with such individuals, was ignoring her body's signals to slow down—signals such as pain, hunger, and fatigue. For the most part, compulsive exercisers work out to burn calories or to lose weight rather than to improve their health or fitness. The thought of missing a workout sends them into a psychological tailspin, often resulting in restricting calories even further, or increasing their exercise the next day. Increased anxiety, depression, or dramatic mood swings can also be signs that an individual's exercise routine is spiraling out of control.

To an eating-disordered individual, exercise can become as addictive as food restricting, bingeing, or purging. And because exercise has been identified as healthful, it can be seen by these individuals as a "legal purge," and obvious warning signals from the body are thus dismissed. Vigorous exercise releases chemicals in the brain that positively affect appetite, sleep, and moods. However, to achieve the desired "high," the compulsive exerciser must exercise more frequently, more intensely, and for longer periods of time.

The dangers inherent in dysfunctional exercise are significant. Teenage girls are particularly at risk, because their nutritional needs are so great and because adolescence is a critical time for the formation of healthy bones. Excessive exercise and/or restrictive dieting can also delay a young woman's normal growth and development. If too much weight is lost, this can lead to cessation of periods and estrogen deficiency, which, together with inadequate calcium and vitamin D intake, puts her at increased risk of adolescent osteoporosis. The consequence of this is very thin, brittle bones that are weblike in consistency. These weak bones lead to a higher risk of stress fractures, in addition to tendon damage and other overuse injuries.

Exercising to the point of exhaustion and then vomiting, like Leslie did, is extremely dangerous. It often results in dehydration, leading to loss of fluids and electrolytes—and even death. Excessive exercise and nutritional deprivation undermine the potential benefit of physical activity: to build muscle and increase fitness levels. Instead, the undernourished body responds by storing fat and burning muscle. This can result in a higher percentage of body fat—the exact *opposite* of what exercise is meant to accomplish. What most people also fail to realize is that without the muscle strength and energy (that is, calories) to work out at their optimum level, they can't burn as many calories as they otherwise would have, because their body is conserving calories to sustain life.

Unfortunately, Leslie's parents seemed out of touch with her disordered behavior, and out of touch with each other as well—a point that is never missed by sensitive teens. If Leslie's parents were more communicative about the apparent stresses their marriage was suffering, Leslie might not have been compelled to "run off" her anxiety or control her eating in such an obsessive and disordered way. If her parents had listened to her concerns about their relationship instead of dismissing her for being dramatic, they might have been able to reassure her that the family's stability was not in jeopardy.

Though parents must retain clear and appropriate privacy boundaries with their adolescent children, it is important that they talk to them about issues and concerns that come up in the family. Communication builds relationships; silence destroys them. If children sense that there is something wrong and nobody's talking, they are prone to imagine that the unspoken problems are even worse then they actually are—and justifiably, they are frightened. Their fear mounts, and yet—because they sense that it's not okay to ask questions—they still can't voice their concerns or seek consolation. As a result, they may turn to unhealthy behaviors to work through their unresolved emotions.

Trying to pretend there is nothing wrong, or that everything is okay when it's not, creates enormous insecurity and stress in children. When parents are willing to listen and talk with their children—no matter how difficult the problem—a safe environment is created, one in which they can share their feelings and concerns. This allows them to cope with all sorts of problems and challenges in healthier ways—further proving how powerful good family communication can be.

CHANGING THE PATTERN

PARENTS

⬡ Be aware if your child has become overly preoccupied with her exercise routine.

⬡ If your child wants to exercise, help her learn to do it properly. Have her consult with the physical education teacher at school, an exercise physiologist, or a certified trainer, who can teach her the importance of a well-rounded routine.

⬡ Support your teen's desire to be active. Exercise together. It's a great way to spend time together and build on your relationship.

TEENS

⬡ Remember that *too much* exercise is hard on your body and can cause stress fractures and other serious medical problems. Regular but moderate exercise has many benefits, as it not only improves physical health but also enhances mood.

⬡ Ask yourself honestly whether you're using exercise as an escape from your troubles. Ask yourself: What am I escaping from? Use your voice. Seek support from parents and professionals who can help you understand and deal with difficult feelings.

≈ Educate yourself about exercise and fitness. In order for your body to be a smooth-running machine, you need to pay attention to your nutrition, which means getting enough calories for your body to operate. Be sure to eat regular meals and snacks, and get plenty of sleep.

SUPPLEMENTARY READING:

FOR PARENTS AND TEENS

The Exercise Balance: What's Too Much, What's Too Little, and What's Just Right for You!, by Pauline Powers and Ron Thompson

Nancy Clark's Sports Nutrition Guidebook, 3rd ed., by Nancy Clark

Scenario 15

MOTHER MAY I?

WHEN PARENTS PROJECT WEIGHT CONCERNS ONTO THEIR TEENS

A mother who radiates self-love and self-acceptance vaccinates her daughter.

—Naomi Wolf

Many parents of overweight children, or children who might become overweight, feel compelled to control their children's eating. In addition to their own worries, parents may receive additional pressure from healthcare providers, schools and teachers, coaches, other family members, and friends.

It is generally believed that fat kids eat too much—and certainly, this is true in some cases. But frequently, overweight children become that way as a result of *underfeeding*. When a parent restricts calories, a child often becomes preoccupied with food and overeats as soon as there is a chance to do so. Though their intentions are good, parents who withhold food may be profoundly interfering with their children's ability to regulate their own eating.

In the following scenario, thirty-nine-year-old Diane desperately wants to save her eleven-year-old daughter, Chelsea, from what she sees as "the scourge" of their family's genetics. She takes matters into her own hands to make sure Chelsea does not become overweight and miss out on going to the prom, like she did.

EVER SINCE I CAN REMEMBER, I'VE BEEN overweight. But when I was twelve, that's when it really started to matter. My sisters and my mother were heavy too, and they all blamed it on genetics. I never believed it—not completely—so I was always trying to lose weight, going on every new diet that came out, each time thinking that maybe *this* was the one. But nothing ever worked! Not only did I regain every pound I lost, I seemed to gain extra weight with each new diet. So recently, I gave in. I resigned myself to being fat for the rest of my life.

But I'm determined that my daughter will *not* have to live like this. Chelsea's twelfth birthday is coming up next month, and she'll be starting middle school soon. That's when everything changes—I know from experience. That's when kids start to get really mean. I refuse to let her be teased and taunted the way I always was! Unlike me, Chelsea *will* have a date for the senior prom. I know that's a long time away, but we have to act now.

Although I know it's frustrating for her, it's my responsibility to train her to eat right. I make sure I know what and how much food is going into her body. And when it comes to extra snacks or second helpings, I tell her that she should drink a glass of water—that will help fill her up, and besides, it's good for the kidneys. I never let her have dessert—I don't even allow them into the house. She can't afford to eat all those empty calories!

But the other day, I found her out. She's been hiding candy in a secret place in the basement—very sneaky. I couldn't believe it! And even though I've asked her friends' parents not to give her food when she goes over to their homes, I suspect they're doing it anyway, because despite my best efforts, Chelsea is gaining a little weight every week. I know the new scale I bought can't be wrong. Doesn't she realize I'm doing this all for her? I wish she would take this seriously. It seems that hiding food and eating behind my back is more like a game to her.

I've suffered all my life because of my weight, and I've tried so hard to make sure Chelsea knows it doesn't have to be the same way for her. I'm completely beside myself. Is my daughter destined to be fat like me?

POINTS TO PONDER

Diane's desire to protect Chelsea from the pain she experienced as an overweight child is very understandable. All parents want to protect their children from being hurt, especially if they have experienced pain and rejection during their own childhoods.

Diane's family history probably did predispose Chelsea to weight problems; studies have shown that genetics do play a role. However, studies have also shown that creating a healthy eating environment and promoting an active lifestyle are even more important than genetics in determining an individual's weight.

Diane's own experience with diets proved that they don't work. Most diets deprive us of necessary calories and limit our food choices. Even more deceptive are the weight-loss programs that promise immediate results, often without exercise. Unfortunately, many people interested in losing weight focus too much on restricting calories, and not enough on exercise.

Without proper information and guidance, most individuals who attempt to lose weight end up doing more harm to their bodies than good, starving themselves instead of better nourishing themselves. The body's reaction to being deprived of necessary calories (and "calories" is just another word for "energy") is a slowdown in metabolism. Severely restricting calories leads to loss of water and muscle weight—not a loss of fat. It may look good on the scale, but this approach prevents *permanent* weight loss, because lean body weight or muscle is lost instead of fat weight. Fat weighs less, but it is also less metabolically active than muscle. When we return to our old eating habits, we're set up to gain even more weight, because there is a higher percentage of fat to lean body weight.

Though well intended, Diane's attempts to monitor Chelsea's eating could lead to harmful consequences. By trying to control Chelsea's food intake, Diane probably created a situation in which her daughter became preoccupied with food and therefore became prone to overeating when she got a chance. By stripping Chelsea of all responsibility relative to her eating behavior, Diane created the environment for Chelsea to become secretive and rebellious.

It is important for parents to provide a variety of good, nutritious food for their children, as well as to establish regular times for meals and snacks. However, allowing children to decide how much they eat —and even whether or not they want to eat —is important. It teaches them to take responsibility for their own food choices, to create their own limits, and to establish a lifelong trust in their body's ability to help them determine their individual hunger and fullness cues. When foods are withheld, they only become more desirable. If children are taught that there are no "good" or "bad" foods, and that *all* foods can be part of a healthy lifestyle, they begin to build a good relationship with food and are empowered with the confidence to eat well.

Early adolescence is an opportune time for children to learn responsibility in all aspects of life, including eating. Parents can offer guidance and support, but they teach most effectively through their own behavior. Had Diane taken a closer look at her own body image and attitude toward food, perhaps she might have found that it wasn't as healthy as it could have been, and realized that before she could help her daughter, she had to help herself. Because changing eating habits and attitudes toward food is difficult at best, seeking professional help from a registered dietitian—who could provide nutritional guidance and support—could have been extremely helpful. A dietitian could have taken an individualized approach to Diane's history and assisted her in making some long-term lifestyle changes—helping her to eat more consciously, to become more aware of serving sizes, and to exercise appropriately. By helping Diane recognize how she might have been using food for emotional reasons, a dietitian could have taught her that "food is meant to nourish, not to nurture." Diane and Chelsea could have benefited greatly, both physically and psychologically, from this kind of work.

Teenagers take nutritional risks because they want to eat like all their friends, *and* because they want to establish their own identities. This is one reason why they benefit greatly from being involved in planning and preparing family meals. Teaching them these kinds of life skills while they are still living at home will enable them to eventually emancipate themselves and get along in the world on their own. By maintaining a positive eating environment and helping children to achieve the body that is right for them, parents allow them to be relaxed and comfortable about eating, and at peace with their bodies.

CHANGING THE PATTERN

PARENTS

⟡   Teach your teen to trust her body's hunger and fullness cues, rather than relying on a diet to tell her what, when, and how to eat.

⟡   Refrain from restricting your child's calorie intake, which can lead to stunted growth, menstrual dysfunction, decreased bone density, and a preoccupation with food.

⟡   Avoid weighing your child. You don't want the number on the scale to determine how they feel about themselves.

⟡   Involve your teen in planning and preparing meals whenever possible. They will be more likely to eat well and will take pride in what they have accomplished.

⟡   Show, by example, how eating *all* foods in moderation can lead to a healthy body and lifestyle.

⟡   Seek professional help from a registered dietitian if your teen is struggling with weight or body image issues. Addressing the problem early can have lifelong benefits.

TEENS

～ Remember: There are no "good" or "bad" foods. All foods can be part of a healthy diet and are meant to be enjoyed.

～ Take responsibility for your own eating. Let your parents know if you aren't getting enough to eat, or if there isn't enough variety to choose from.

～ If you sense you are beginning to use food for comfort, or are becoming preoccupied with food, let your parents know. Consider seeing a dietitian to help you change the way you think about food; this will lead to lifelong health and fitness.

～ Don't despair: Even if you are genetically predisposed to being overweight, there are plenty of ways to stay healthy and feel great about yourself. A healthy attitude about food and regular exercise has a much bigger and better influence on your health, fitness, and mood than dieting.

Scenario 16

LENGTHENING THE LEASH

WHEN A CLOSE RELATIONSHIP
IS TOO CLOSE

When a father gives his daughter an emotional visa to strike out on her own, he is always with her. Such a daughter has her encouraging, understanding daddy in her head, cheering her on—not simply as a woman, but as a whole, unique human being with unlimited possibilities.

—Victoria Secunda

A sense of independence, age-appropriate expectations, and healthy boundaries allow teenagers to grow and find their own internal strengths. So when parents are overprotective or overinvolved in their children's lives, their children may feel smothered and unable to make the important transition to adulthood. Throughout their childhood and teen years, it is normal and natural for the division of responsibility between parent and child to change. As children grow and mature, they begin to take on more responsibility for themselves and their decisions. To encourage that shift in responsibility is to forge a relationship built on mutual respect and trust, and parents who do so can enjoy the wonderful experience of helping their children grow into decisive and competent adults.

In this scenario, thirteen-year-old Hanna and her father share a very close, loving relationship. However, when Hanna starts going to middle school and wants more independence, her dad puts on the brakes.

EVERYONE ALWAYS TELLS ME HOW LUCKY I

am. My dad does everything for me. As he puts it, I'm the apple of his eye. He picks me up from school in his shiny new Cadillac every day, and he always makes a big deal about opening the door for me, saying, "Your highness." He brags to everyone about his "pretty little princess" and tells them how proud he is of me. That's why I try so hard to be the very best in school and at Pony Club. No way can I let him down after all he's built up about me!

I was even more worried than usual about this stuff when I started middle school, which seemed so big compared to grade school. There were so many kids! I knew it was going to be very different. It was a little scary at first, and being shy didn't help. I never had many friends anyway. But I didn't really feel like I needed lots of friends. I always had so much fun with my family. I just tried to remember how Mom told me about how shy she had been at my age, and how she had concentrated on making just one friend at a time. When I thought about it that way, it didn't seem so scary.

I think it's working too. I already made one good friend, Beth. And at lunch today, a couple of girls asked me to join them. Plus, Jeremy—who's *really* cute—asked me if he could call me tonight!

I couldn't wait to tell Dad about my new friends, and especially about Jeremy. But when I mentioned Jeremy's name, he snapped at me, saying "You're too young to be thinking about boys." When he saw my face though, he smiled and hugged me, saying, "Besides, aren't I your guy? You and I are buddies, remember?" I just looked at my feet and said, "Sorry, Dad. I didn't mean to hurt your feelings."

I know how much he loves me, and I would never want to make him sad, but I couldn't help feeling angry. I really like Jeremy, and I really want him to call me! I would have asked Mom about it if I thought it would help at all, but Dad's opinion always seems to overpower hers. She doesn't even seem to try anymore. And lately, she even seems kind of mad about my relationship with Dad, calling me a "Daddy's girl" or making fun of how I look or what I'm wearing. It kind of feels like she's jealous of me. I can't imagine why. But now that I think of it, I can't remember the last time I saw Mom and Dad hug or show any affection to each other.

That night when Jeremy called, Dad answered the phone and made some lame excuse as to why I couldn't talk. I was really angry, because I like Jeremy and wanted to talk to him. I wish Dad would realize that I'm growing up, and that it's kind of fun having a boy interested in me. Sure, boys can be dorky, but Jeremy's different. But then again, Dad always seems to know what is right, and he's always looking out for me. I just didn't understand why I felt so awful about it. I was so confused. I pretended to have a stomachache at dinner so I wouldn't have to sit there and eat and go through the routine of answering all Dad's questions about my day while Mom just ate her food in silence. The thought of it made me want to *scream*. I just wanted to be left alone, to have some time to think—some privacy!

When I got to my bedroom, I flung myself onto my bed and sobbed quietly into my pillow. *Am I ever going to be able to do anything without Dad sticking his big nose into it?* I wondered. I'm not a little kid anymore. I don't know why I'm still being treated like one.

Don't get me wrong. I love my dad. He's the greatest. But I want to spend more time with my friends. I know how much he loves me, but I'm getting too old for him to pick me up from school every day. I'd rather take the bus home with my friends. I used to love sitting on the sofa and cuddling with him, but I'm too old for that too. I just don't know how to tell him how I feel.

I haven't told anyone yet—especially not Mom or Dad—but tonight wasn't the first time I skipped a meal. I'm not sure when it really started, but I think it's been going on for a few weeks now. What I figured out is that when I'm really upset, and don't eat, I think about food, and not about how upset I am. I don't know how, but it seems to work. I guess it kind of helps me not to feel so guilty about being angry at Mom and Dad. It seems like I'm more in control of at least something in my life. After all, no one can force me to eat if I don't want to.

POINTS TO PONDER

Though he may have felt that he was only showing his daughter love and protection, Hanna's father was controlling most every aspect of his daughter's life. At this stage of development, the main task of the early adolescent is to gain autonomy from their parents and to focus on peers—in other words, to learn how to be a part of the teenage world.

This can be a difficult transition for both teens and parents. Parents most likely have had a hands-on relationship with their child up to this point. Starting to let go can be a scary but necessary step in allowing teenagers to grow up and discover who they are. As was illustrated in this scenario, Hanna felt so sheltered and controlled by her dad that she unwittingly developed an eating disorder as a way of finding some independence and control in her life.

Hanna's father seemed to be very fulfilled by his intimacy with his daughter—probably to an unhealthy degree. Intimacy between him and his wife seemed to be lacking or even nonexistent. In addition, Hanna's relationship with her parents was dominated by her father's presence, and her relationship with her mother suffered because of this. The imbalance of the father-daughter relationship may have made Hanna's mother feel powerless and inadequate. Starting to see her own daughter as a rival for her husband's affection, Hanna's mother began to be critical and demeaning toward Hanna. This type of behavior could be extremely destructive to Hanna's relationship with her mother.

The absence of a strong female role model can be difficult for a young woman, because such a woman can show her how to set good boundaries and tell her that she has the right to say *no* to something she is uncomfortable with. If Hanna had such a role model in her mother, she might have been more comfortable standing up to her father and discontinuing the probably inappropriate cuddling with him. She might have been able to disregard his forbiddance of her phone call with Jeremy, or to turn to her mother for support.

Although the mother's role is important to an adolescent girl, it is a natural part of the developmental process for a young woman to pull away from her dependency on her mother, and to look to her father to teach her about the outside world. Fathers play a significant role in helping their daughters transition from childhood to becoming a young woman. Unfortunately, many men feel ill-equipped or uncomfortable relating to their teenage daughters as they watch them mature and become more sexual.

To an adolescent girl, her father is the most important man in her life. When a dad is able to help his daughter feel attractive and acceptable in a nonsexual way, he enables her to accept her changing body and develop the confidence to relate to the opposite sex. However, when this acceptance does not occur, for whatever reason, many young girls experience self-doubt and depression. They are unable to develop a comfort level with their more womanly shape and may withdraw from social interactions, become promiscuous, and have less of a sense of self. A young girl's inability to accept her changing body or her desire to maintain a more childlike physique can be expressed through an eating disorder.

A strong marital bond provides the safety within which a young girl can grow and learn to appreciate what a healthy relationship between a man and a woman looks like. If the marriage is shaky, or if Mom and Dad are fighting constantly, the child often lives in fear that one or the other parent will leave. Even more damaging to the child's self-worth is the fact that she often begins to blame herself for the problems that exist between her parents. Perhaps she feels that it is up to her to fix them. In order not to create any waves, young girls growing up in this environment often attempt to be "perfect" and deny their own needs.

Both mothers and fathers play a critical role in helping their daughters define themselves. Both are instrumental in teaching young women how to make conscious choices and set good boundaries. By showing a daughter that her opinions are respected and valued, parents can help her develop her sense of self and build a strong character. Encouraging a daughter to stand up for herself, and allowing her to set limits on her time, her activities, and her friends can give her the confidence to trust her own judgment and establish her own set of values and goals. Parents should not miss the opportunity to form this sacred bond with their daughter as she prepares to enter adolescence and— with parental guidance—grow into a strong, well-adjusted young woman.

CHANGING THE PATTERN

PARENTS

❧   Allow your teen some independence when appropriate. It helps them to develop trust in themselves and their ability to make good decisions.

❧   If you suspect that an adult or parent is being overly intimate or inappropriate, take action immediately to rectify the situation. As a parent, you are your child's most important ally.

❧   Spend time with your teen. When you have a strong parent-child bond, you will be the first one they seek out when a problem comes up.

❧   Spend time alone with your spouse—without the kids. Nurture and value that important relationship.

TEENS

❦ Stand up for yourself. Express your needs clearly and lovingly to your parents, and try to explain why these things are important to you.

❦ Listen to your feelings. Put a voice to how you feel. It can help you from going underground with your feelings and developing unhealthy coping behaviors.

❦ Tell a trusted adult if you feel an adult or parent is behaving with you in an inappropriate way. It is *not* a betrayal for you to take care of yourself. See below for information on how to get help.

SUPPLEMENTARY READING AND RESOURCES:

FOR PARENTS

Father Hunger: Fathers, Daughters, and the Pursuit of Thinness, by Margo Maine

FOR TEENS

National Sexual Assault Hotline (totally confidential): 1-800-656-HOPE (4673)

RAINN (Rape, Abuse & Incest National Network)
www.rainn.org
America's largest anti–sexual assault organization

Teen Help

www.teenhelp.com

Information for teens, parents, and other adults on issues such as eating disorders, pregnancy, sexual abuse, suicide, depression, and stress

Scenario 17

A WELL-STOCKED PANTRY

WHEN A TEEN NEEDS
MORE FOOD CHOICES

If you are not free to choose wrongly and irresponsibly, you are not free at all.

—Jacob Hornberger

Healthy choices nourish the mind, body, and spirit. This is true of the activities we choose to participate in, as well as the foods we choose to eat. Parents play a key role in what food choices are available in the home, since they are generally responsible for doing the grocery shopping. They also are instrumental in creating an atmosphere in the home that helps their children develop a positive relationship with food.

When parents diet—and restrict what foods they allow into the house to avoid being tempted by "forbidden foods," or when they purchase only foods allowed on their diet—they set up a dangerous dynamic. They not only compromise their own health, but also the health of the rest of the family. Teens are especially at risk in such a situation, because their nutritional needs are so great.

In the following scenario, eighteen-year-old Sarah is the star volleyball player on her high school team. She comes home after practice feeling extremely hungry, only to find very little food in the house because of her mother's new diet.

VOLLEYBALL SEASON IS IN FULL SWING, AND

Coach Hunter is working us really hard. He's hoping to get us to the state championships again this year—after all, it's a school tradition. Since I'm a senior and the starting setter on the team, I'm really feeling the pressure. Not just from my coach, but from the entire school. Everyone seems to be counting on me. I love volleyball, and I want to win just as much as everyone else—probably more, actually! But there's no doubt: We have a very tough season ahead of us.

All this was racing through my mind as I came home after practice today. I threw my jacket on the kitchen chair and went straight to the fridge. We'd had a really hard practice, and I was absolutely starving. But what did I find? Nothing—except for a tub of disgusting cottage cheese and Mom's leftover steak from last night. It made me want to scream! Mom started this new protein-only diet, and now there aren't any normal foods in the house. She's always dieting, and our kitchen is littered with weight-loss books, weird gross shakes in a can, and powders and pills that she adds to her diets. It really bothers me. But then, to make matters worse, she got rid of most of the stuff I like to eat when she decided last month that she's "addicted to carbs." She said she wanted to clear the house of any "temptations." Now there's not even bread for me to make toast, or a peanut butter and jelly sandwich!

A couple weeks ago, I tried to talk to my mom about how her dieting is affecting me and the rest of the family, but it's like she couldn't even hear what I was trying to say. She just zoned out. All she can think about is how she looks, and losing weight. I'm really worried about her. She told me once that her dad was always hard on her because she tended to be on the chunky side. Maybe that's why she's so hard on herself.

Knowing that volleyball season was about to start, and remembering how hungry I always felt after practice last year, I thought it might be helpful if I gave her a list of foods to buy for me at the grocery store. That way she wouldn't have to think about it. But she said she didn't even want to have to *look* for those foods in the store, because now she only went to the meat counter, and going down any of the other grocery store aisles would just make it harder for her to stick to her diet. Instead, she just gave me some money so I could buy lunch at school or pick up some food on the way home. Who has time for that?

When I saw that there was nothing to eat in the fridge, I slammed the door shut and yelled out, "Why can't we ever have anything decent to eat in this house?" But no one was home to hear me. Mom wasn't home from work yet, and my little sister was probably next door playing with her friend. I was so hungry I felt like I was going to pass out. Suddenly I remembered that my sister still had a stash of Halloween candy under her bed. I ran upstairs, got the bag, and—like an animal—stuffed ten little candy bars into my face. Within minutes, I felt sick to my stomach. And of course, the guilt and anxiety flooded in. Ten candy bars! I'm going to get fat and gross and look disgusting in my volleyball shorts! I ran to the bathroom and stuck my finger down my throat.

Now, I'm beginning to worry about *me* too—not just Mom. When I get that hungry, I eat whatever I can get my hands on. And it seems to be happening more and more. But I can't afford to gain weight, so the only thing I can do is get rid of it. With the team depending on me, I've got to eat, or I'm going to wind up passing out or being too weak to play. I don't know what to do.

POINTS TO PONDER

There are a few important factors to consider here. The most obvious is that Sarah had no control of her food choices. Second, no one was home when Sarah got home from practice—which is normal and typical in today's world. It is not a problem in and of itself when an adult isn't at home after school, but it may have been that Sarah did not yet have the tools and experience to figure things out on her own, without the support of her parents. If she'd had more time to spend with her parents, she might have found a way to express her needs, to be listened to, and to problem-solve with them. Third, Sarah's mother was setting a harmful precedent for both of her daughters by always being on a diet. She was showing, by example, that she was unable to manage her own food choices and weight. In addition to conveying that she didn't trust her body enough to know what and how much to eat, she was perhaps setting the stage for the girls to engage in unhealthy eating practices or behaviors themselves.

Like all women in our society, young girls are under tremendous pressure to possess the perfect body and to be thin at all costs. Women have been encouraged to view their bodies as ornamental rather than functional. Even in sports—where we would hope young girls would receive positive affirmations about their bodies—they are often under unrealistic expectations to "look good" rather than being admired for their athletic abilities. We saw this with Sarah: Although she was a star athlete at school, she seemed to be more concerned with how she looked in her volleyball shorts than how she would perform in the upcoming matches.

Inherent in all high school sports are the increased demands on the student athlete. Most coaches require daily practices or scheduled games after school. This limits the time students have for homework and social interaction with friends who aren't their teammates. Time with the family can be very fragmented, and sitting down together for a meal becomes almost impossible—especially if the parents are very busy too. As a result, high school athletes often find themselves emotionally and physically exhausted.

High school is a time of tremendous growth spurts for teens, and they need to fuel their bodies to meet those demands. Second only to infancy, adolescence is the fastest growth stage of life, and all too often, teen years can be a time when food choices *aren't* compatible with nutritional needs. Recognizing this fact, parents play an important role in ensuring that their teens eat regular meals and snacks. Making sure that food is available in sufficient quantities to meet their children's growing caloric needs provides teenagers with a feeling of safety and assurance that there will always be enough to eat.

Both teenage girls and boys experience a normal increase in appetite because of their body's increased calorie needs for growth and development. But because most adolescent girls are already worried about gaining weight, it is extremely important that they have access to a good variety of healthy, nutritious foods. This lessens their anxiety and ensures that they have plenty of choices to satisfy their hunger.

Nutrition is critical during the teen years—not only because of growth and development, but because teens are laying the groundwork for their adult eating habits. That's why it's so important for parents to be good role models. Diets almost never work—studies show that they fail 90 to 95 percent of the time.

Parents can set an example for healthy eating by eating well themselves. Instead of depriving themselves, they would do well to use a more sensible approach that includes exercise and cutting back on portion sizes. By adopting a healthier lifestyle and losing weight gradually, adults are more likely to keep it off for life, in addition to setting a good example for their teens.

Some basic rules to follow would be to eat at least three meals a day and, depending on activity level, to incorporate nutritious snacks as well. Having a good variety of foods (grains, fruits and vegetables, meats, poultry and fish, milk and dairy products, and healthy fats) allows an individual to get all the nutrients he or she needs, and to avoid the boredom that occurs when following a restrictive diet. Some examples of nutritious snacks are fruit smoothies, veggies and dip, sliced apples and bananas, cheese and crackers, or a bean burrito.

Family meals—during which the parents' example is readily seen and experienced—are a good idea. In today's busy households, it may not be possible to eat together every night, but scheduling three to four dinners a week should do the trick. The family meal also provides an excellent opportunity for parents and teens to touch base about what's going on in their lives, and about how they're feeling in general. Communication within the family, and spending quality time together, can help both parents and teens get their needs met, in addition to building on their relationships. Should issues arise, the strong bond that has been forged allows for open and honest discussion, and a resolution of problems before they get out of control.

CHANGING THE PATTERN

PARENTS

~ Quit dieting. It doesn't work, and it's not setting a good example for your teen. If you have weight concerns, instead adopt a healthier lifestyle that includes exercise.

~ Keep plenty of healthy food choices in the house. Teens need extra energy and nutrition while they are developing.

~ Talk to your teen to find out what kind of foods they would like to have available. Keep a grocery list handy that they can add to. This allows them to take some responsibility for their own food choices.

~ Plan meals and snacks with your teen. This is a great time to set a good example of healthy eating choices.

~ Set a goal of three to four dinners together each week. Family mealtime is critical to good nutrition and communication.

TEENS

~ Talk to your parents if you feel there are not enough food choices for you at home. Tell them it's important for you to eat well and often while you are growing.

❧ Know that it's healthy and normal for you to have a bigger appetite during this time—especially if you're an athlete. Your body needs extra energy right now.

❧ Speak up and let your parents know if you are concerned about them. Stuffing your feelings down and not talking about them can hurt you. Trust your instincts.

Scenario 18

LEAVING HOME

WHEN A TEEN GOES
OFF TO COLLEGE

Leaving home in a sense involves a kind of second birth in which we give birth to ourselves.

—Robert Neelly Bellah

A common time for an eating disorder to erupt in a young girl's life is during her senior year in high school. The realization hits that she has to grow up and face all of the challenges of leaving home and entering college—academics, dating, fitting in, dealing with choices about alcohol and drugs, living in a dorm, and not having parents to sit with and talk to when things don't go well.

For a teen who's afraid of facing these challenges, the prospect of going off on her own and becoming more independent is terrifying, because it means making tough choices by herself—and taking responsibility for those choices. Often there is an unconscious desire to stay young and not become more mature. An anorexic body—thin and straight—is an expression of this fear of maturity. If a girl is able to look younger than her actual years, she may think she can escape the adult responsibilities that come with college and becoming independent.

This underlying issue can manifest itself in the fear of dealing with the "Freshman 15," a common myth that students gain fifteen pounds when confronted with dorm food. Some high school seniors, fearful of this myth, try to head off the problem by losing weight before leaving for college. If a girl gets skinny enough before she leaves, then she feels fortified against the feared weight before she ever leaves home. In fact, she may unconsciously realize that if she loses enough weight, maybe she won't be well enough to leave home at all.

Much of these thought processes, whether conscious or not, are a way to deal with a reluctance to leave childhood and face the world as a mature adult. The food concerns seem to have a simpler and more concrete resolution and mask the more deeply seated issue of facing the separation from home and parents. With a measurable focus on pounds lost, anxiety subsides, and energy goes toward accomplishing a tangible goal that *seems* like the real problem but is actually a red herring and solves nothing.

In the next scenario, seventeen-year-old Danielle faces her college applications and realizes that she is afraid to leave home.

I STARED AT THE COLLEGE APPLICATIONS

spread out before me on the kitchen table and felt sick to my stomach. I just wanted to rip them up and run to my room. It was all too much, and a million thoughts and worries were plaguing me. I didn't want to leave home. But all of my friends were applying to colleges out of state. I couldn't understand why they wanted to go so far away. What was wrong with the state university? The thought of college *anywhere* was scary enough, but all the way across the *country*?

I didn't want to be different from everyone else, but I guess I was, because I couldn't face the thought of being so far away that I couldn't go home on weekends if I felt homesick. *Is there something wrong with me?* I wondered. *How come my friends are braver than I am?*

To make matters worse, I couldn't think of anyone I could talk to about it. Not even my best friend, Sara. She was applying at one of the big ten and would probably get in. She didn't seem scared at all. My brother and I were pretty close, but he was only a sophomore in high school and wasn't even thinking about college yet. How could he help? I didn't want to tell my parents and dash all of their hopes about my future. That wouldn't be fair. I couldn't think of one person who could understand and not judge me for being scared of something as silly as going to college.

Just a few months ago, college sounded exciting. But I guess the reality of it had finally sunk in. And there were so many unknowns. What would the kids be like? Who would I talk to when I was upset? Would anybody like me? What if I hated dorm food and gained tons of weight? These thoughts terrified me.

I stared at the mess of applications and wondered how I could ever write the required essays about why I should be accepted at schools I didn't even want to go to. I'd visited most of them last summer with my parents. Back then, they looked exciting, and I couldn't wait until it was my turn to go. Now the memories of the beautiful campuses and ivy-covered buildings made me wonder what I'd been thinking. At the time, I'd told my parents that I couldn't *wait* to go, and now I couldn't think of a way to bow out gracefully. Mom and Dad had no idea that I was filled with dread, and they were making daily comments about how exciting it must be to be thinking about college.

I put my head in my hands and restrained myself from ripping up the applications. I wondered why I'd waited until the last minute to work on them. *Why does this have to be so hard? I just want to stay in high school forever,* I thought. But I didn't have one friend who was staying here next year. Besides, I'd never get out of going. My parents would kill me and think I was being a baby. *Why didn't someone warn me that I would have these feelings?*

My mind raced as I tried to think of a way to get out of leaving without letting anyone know that I was having these thoughts. A solution seemed impossible. And then I thought about my friend Kathy, and that made it worse. Kathy had gone off to college last year and put on the famous "Freshman

15." She used to be skinny and beautiful. When she came home for winter break, she was still pretty, but she'd really gained a lot of weight that first semester. *I would die if that happened to me,* I thought. I knew that my parents would never let me live off campus, where I wouldn't have to deal with dorm food. They just didn't have the money to rent me an apartment or to help me buy the kind of food I thought was safe. I knew I would be stuck with the starchy stuff that dorm cafeterias always served. *No way*, I thought. *I cannot let that happen to me.*

Then it occurred to me: *It doesn't have to happen to me. In fact, it won't happen to me. This is fixable*, I thought. *I will lose just enough before I go so that if I gain fifteen pounds, it won't matter.* Now was obviously the time to get started on a diet—way before I ever got there. I was determined not to end up like Kathy, and I made a solemn vow to start my diet the next day. How hard could it be? Hadn't I always been able to accomplish anything I really set as a goal? Easy. I knew I could look on the Internet and find any diet information I needed, and I would do that research after I finished all of these applications, which suddenly seemed manageable.

I let out a sigh of relief and picked up the first application. I decided to do this essay on paper and then type it up on my computer, after I had given it some thought. The words flowed as I wrote about my desire to be a part of their student body, and how their course of study fit my career goals. I wrote eloquently about how I could contribute to the campus newspaper and play my viola in the orchestra. College didn't sound so bad now. In fact, I thought this one *was* probably my first choice. When I visited the campus, the kids seemed friendly. I hoped I would get an early acceptance and have it all settled.

The dieting was easier than I thought it would be. In fact, I was exhilarated after the first few days of giving up sweets and sodas. I loved the clean feeling of having my body slim down pound after pound, day after day. Coffee was helping me to keep my energy going, and salads became my friends. Nothing could stop this pursuit of thinness, and I wondered why I hadn't tried this sooner. My friends began to notice the change in how I looked, and the compliments from my parents felt good. By graduation, I couldn't imagine why I had ever worried about college. I could hardly wait for the summer to be over so I could get there and make an appearance as the new, much slimmer Danielle.

It wasn't too long before I lost fifteen pounds, but I felt so proud and looked so good that I kept going, all the way down to eighty-five pounds. But soon my periods stopped, and just one month before I was supposed to leave, my parents got worried and took me to the doctor, who said I was too thin and that I had to stay at the hospital.

I hate the hospital. It's awful here. And to make matters worse, the doctor said my blood work was so messed up that I'm too sick to go to college. My parents sided with the doctor and wouldn't let me go.

"How can you *do* this!" I shouted. "I've been accepted at my first-choice school!" But no amount of shouting made a difference.

Now all my friends have left for college, and I'm still in the hospital. I'm absolutely devastated. It's so unfair! I worked so hard and was successful with my diet. And I wasn't afraid of college anymore. I *wanted* to go! But the doctor and my parents are all saying that I have to gain weight back until I have reached what *they* call a healthy number on the scale. Don't they understand how much better I feel like this? I would hate myself if I got bigger and looked like I did before. I never want to see all that weight on my body again.

POINTS TO PONDER

Senior year in high school is a time when anorexia can serve as a crystallized way to quell the anxiety that can overwhelm teens who fear maturity. In the beginning of the scenario, Danielle was dealing with the fear of separation and emancipation that often comes with the prospect of going to college. In the process of completing her applications, she felt very overwhelmed and out of control. Once Danielle became aware of her fears, she was further troubled by the belief that she had no one to discuss those fears with. Although she apparently never actually asked any other girls, she assumed she was the only one among her circle of friends who had these concerns. In all likelihood, many if not most of her friends had a similar sense of anxiety, but because she was too embarrassed to admit her own worries, she never shared them with anyone, and never found out that she was not alone.

She searched her mind for a solution that would not disappoint her parents and would not require her to reveal the shame she felt about being afraid. Eventually, she landed on the idea of starting a diet that would make her thin enough to face college with confidence and peace of mind. The idea of dieting and losing weight consoled her, because she believed she now had a concrete way to reassure herself that she would be popular and would not become overweight. She had a way to feel in control.

Danielle obviously enjoyed her home and saw it as a comforting place; otherwise, she probably would not have been worried about leaving. However, we have to wonder why Danielle did not feel okay about turning to her parents for support. Did she feel they could not handle her emotions? Did she feel pressured to please them? Were they both too busy with work and other concerns to be in touch with her fears, or to notice earlier how thin she was getting? If her parents were able to stay more tuned in to her feelings or had noticed her weight loss sooner, they could have encouraged her to talk freely and find a healthier solution than the anorexic direction that prevented her from leaving for college.

We also don't know why Danielle was so afraid of growing up. It could be that Danielle was just born with a fearful temperament and simply needed her parents' understanding. Or her parents might have had their own unconscious reasons for not wanting her to leave, and the reasons affected Danielle unconsciously. This can happen if a couple's marriage is in trouble, because the teen's departure would force them to face their own problems. Sometimes it can happen when parents are insecure and need to have a child around to feel more grown-up themselves. Whether or not Danielle's parents played an active role in the problem, they could have been more observant and encouraged better communication with her as she began to show signs of anorexia.

Danielle could have voiced her fears more freely as well. She was seventeen years old and could have initiated a conversation that might have led to more support from her family, assuaged her anxiety, and helped her to use different coping mechanisms to approach this new stage in her independence. The anorexia may have been saying what she was having trouble putting into words more directly. Finding her voice could have taken away the need to speak through the eating disorder's symptoms.

If her parents could have understood the *real* issue—the fear of growing up—they could have worked together as a family to find a solution that made the eating disorder unnecessary. For example, maybe Danielle needed another year of maturity before she left for college, or at least a year at a local junior college, to make the transition smoother and less scary. Maybe a discussion about the "Freshman 15" could have relieved that fear and led to a conversation about healthy eating in a dorm atmosphere. Regardless of the ultimate solution, Danielle would have benefited from an open conversation about the process of leaving home.

Parents need to understand what a huge step it is for a teen to leave home and go to college. They should be on the lookout for signs of distress or unusual behavior, such as extreme weight loss. They also need to examine their own reactions to the process, as it is a transition for parents as well as teens. Open communication in the family sets the stage for a smooth transition for everyone and may avert the need for an eating disorder.

CHANGING THE PATTERN

PARENTS

❧ Be aware of your teen's reactions to the process of preparing to leave home. Don't miss the subtle signs.

❧ Keep the lines of communication open as your teen prepares to leave for college. She may be afraid to tell you that she has fears, and may need you to bring about a conversation that makes it safe for her to talk about her feelings.

❧ Check in with your own emotions when a child is about to leave home. Discuss your own anxiety about her departure with your spouse or with a counselor.

❧ If symptoms arise as your teen prepares to leave, bring up your concerns to her and find help before she is in the grips of a full-blown disorder.

TEENS

✎ Recognize that going away to college is a big step in your development toward adulthood. Some anxiety about the process is understandable. There is nothing shameful about feeling vulnerable in the face of new challenges.

✎ Don't be afraid to air your fears with your parents or other trusted adults. Talking about your feelings always adds perspective to a scary situation and makes it seem more manageable.

✎ Remember that extreme weight loss is not a solution to feeling more confident when you leave home. Drastic dieting can lead to an eating disorder that makes you feel worse about yourself in the long run and prevents you from enjoying the independence that you will gradually embrace as you grow up.

Scenario 19

THE SUPERMODEL SEDUCTION

WHEN THE BRAINWASHING BEGINS

Ours is a society obsessed by weight. In what is surely a crime against innocence, we have set a monster loose among our children. How can we get the monster back in the bottle?
—Frances Berg

At increasingly younger ages, girls—and now, boys—are being affected by society's obsession with thinness and the desire to have "the perfect body." Our media and culture foster the idea that in order to be successful, happy, or virtuous, you must be thin—and those who don't meet the body-size criteria must be lazy, self-indulgent, and out of control. The pressure to meet such unrealistic goals is bound to have significant ramifications on children, who as a result may grow up to be food-phobic, and may judge themselves and others based on outward appearances.

Unfortunately, parents and their children are more likely to learn about nutrition and food from television and magazines (that is, from advertisers trying to sell products) than from dietitians and other health professionals who actually *do* care about their clients' health and well-being. As a result, society's image of physical perfection and ideas about proper nutrition are dictated by the whims of corporations and Hollywood, whose true interests are in making a buck.

In the following scenario, twelve-year-old Cindy is so taken with the models in fashion magazines that she can't think of anything else she would rather be, and she'll go to great lengths to make sure her dream comes true.

JENNIFER IS MY BEST FRIEND IN THE WHOLE

world. I can't remember ever not knowing her! We've grown up together in the same neighborhood, and we basically spend all of our time together. When we were little, we used to play Barbies every single day. We'd spend hours changing our Barbies' clothes and dressing them up in the bajillions of outfits we collected, and we'd make up stories about their adventurous and romantic lives with their handsome boy-friends. We even custom-decorated Jennifer's Barbie Dream House. I remember we used to talk on and on about how we wished we could be just like Barbie when we grew up.

But now we're in seventh grade, so we're over that kid stuff, of course. Now we just hang out in our bedrooms and look at fashion magazines. We like to find pictures of our favorite models and cut them out to put them on our bedroom walls, like a collage. It takes a long time, but it's totally worth it. It looks so cool, and having our idols on our walls all the time helps to inspire us. Sometimes we'll take turns finding a model that looks the most like one of us, or models we think we could be prettier than—if we only had professional makeup artists and cool clothes and stuff. And now there's this new TV show that we absolutely love. It's about all these girls trying to become supermodels, and what their lives are like. They are so glamorous, and they get to go to all these exotic places for their photo shoots. What an amazing life they must have. I want to be exactly like them. I can't wait to grow up and have a sexy body and wear some of those awesome hot outfits.

School is okay, but besides Jennifer, the other girls all seem totally immature. I couldn't care less about the lame boys at our school, or about participating in school activities. But then Jennifer goes and decides to join the school choir. I couldn't believe it! She wanted me to join too, but I'm not into singing. I didn't think she was either. It seems totally dorky and childish. I don't know what's gotten into her. I thought we had bigger plans. When I asked her why she would do something like that without talking to me first, she said her mom made her. But I'm not so sure. She actually seems to be enjoying it, and now she's hanging out with some of the girls in the choir. I feel kind of left out, but I'm not giving up my dream.

My mom's been bugging me to join a club or start playing some kind of musical instrument or sport, but I'm not interested in that stuff, and I'm definitely not going to risk getting too muscular. I know I can't afford to sit around and get fat, though, either. I've got to keep up with an exercise routine. If I don't, it could totally ruin my chances to become a model. But my mom says going to a gym is not enough. She says I have to *do* something, with *people.* She's been relentless.

The other day she suggested that I try out for the school play. I thought about it, but I'm not big on getting up in front of people—maybe I should practice that, though, because models have to do that all the time. It might be good experience—as long as it helps me achieve my true destiny. I just wish Jennifer would do it with me, but she said she's too busy with choir practice. She's not being much of a friend these days. Where is she when I need her?

Oh, well, whether Jennifer wants to join me or not, I'm not giving up on my goal. Every day I make sure to spend time looking at my body in the mirror to see where I can improve. Sometimes it's my arms that look too fat; sometimes it's my ankles. I noticed the other day that my teeth weren't as white as they should be. It's hard to do this critique all by myself though. I really wish I had an outsider's point of view, but Jennifer's spending so much time doing choir stuff now that this daily mirror check is something that I invented and decided to do all by myself.

I'm really beginning to feel like I'm all alone, and even when Jennifer and I do get together, which isn't very often, we are starting to argue. That *never* used to happen. We always thought alike—or at least I thought we did. But yesterday, she got totally annoyed with me because I told her I didn't want to eat microwave popcorn anymore. It used to be part of our ritual, but when I looked at the box and saw how many calories are in it, I was horrified. She sneered at me and said, "Cindy, it's fat-free." That's when I realized that I can't ever tell her about my new diet. She would think I was losing it. And she might even tell my mom.

The diet I'm on now is the hardest one I've ever tried, but from everything I've read, it promises the best results: a perfect body. The instructions on the back of the bottle said I should use it in place of one meal per day, but I'm going to reach my goal weight as quickly as possible, so I'm drinking it twice a day and fasting every other day. Like I said, it's hard, but it's getting easier. The tricky part is how to make sure I can keep the fact that I'm dieting a secret from Mom—and now, apparently, from Jennifer. I know they would try to get in the way. They just don't understand how important this is to me, and that this is what I need to do if I'm ever going to get discovered by an agent.

POINTS TO PONDER

Cindy lived in a fantasy world, based at first on Barbie dolls, and then on fashion magazines and the media's ideal of feminine beauty. She and Jennifer were mesmerized by the good-looking people, outfits, and accessories they saw in their magazines, interpreting what they saw as the perfect life. Cindy, in particular, began to lose interest in all other pursuits, and to totally focus on trying to fit into that fantasy world. Although Cindy's mother was apparently gaining awareness of some of her daughter's developing problems, and was trying to encourage a more active social life, she didn't yet seem to be aware of Cindy's plans to lose weight.

It's tough for parents to know things like this, especially when teens are being secretive. That's why a relationship built on mutual respect and trust—coupled with frequent deep conversations about how the teen is feeling—is so very important for catching or averting the development of an eating disorder. In addition to encouraging Cindy to participate in a social activity, some serious talks needed to take place—talks about nutrition, about advertising, and about emotions.

While Cindy's parents did not necessarily need to discourage her from becoming a model, if that's what she truly wished, they might have been able to broaden her horizons. After all, it was clear that Cindy had spent so much time with her nose in fashion magazines that she had blinders on to becoming anything other than a model. Because she was limiting her everyday experiences, she probably didn't even see that she had many other talents that could provide her with an exciting and exotic life. By having regular conversations about her many talents and possibilities, Cindy's parents may have been able to encourage her to try new things and get her excited about other career paths, in addition to modeling.

Most young girls are fascinated by the fashion industry and enjoy flipping through magazines, looking at the latest styles or getting fashion tips, and reading about the lives of their favorite celebrities or music idols. It is perfectly normal for them to be curious about the culture they are becoming a part of. However, if they are spending too much of their free time with TV, the Internet, and magazines—where the messages is "You need to be prettier; you need to be skinnier"—their view of themselves can become very narrow, and they may develop a limited idea of what they are capable of accomplishing.

Girls—and now boys too—are being affected by this obsession with thinness at increasingly younger ages. The media's idea of beauty is extremely influential, effectively brainwashing our youth when they are most impressionable, and setting them up with completely unrealistic and damaging expectations. Carolyn Costin expressed appropriate alarm at some very disturbing statistics in her book *The Eating Disorder Sourcebook:*

What does it mean when studies show that 95 percent of American women report disgust or disappointment with their bodies? When fashion models are 23 percent below normal weight? When adolescent girls are snorting cocaine, not to get high but to lose weight? When 70 to 80 percent of fourth-grade girls are dieting and claim they would rather be dead than fat?

It is difficult, but very possible, for parents to offset the influence the culture and the media have on their teenagers. By limiting exposure to insidious advertising, parents can redirect their teens' interests toward activities and creative endeavors that help them grow into healthy and productive adults. Also, it is a very good idea to have a frank talk, with both boys and girls, about the agenda of advertisers, and about the unreality of what is being presented to them. An excellent resource to learn more about this important issue is through Dove's Campaign for Real Beauty. The website affiliated with the campaign (www.campaignforrealbeauty.com) informs visitors how much advertisers create impossible standards, and offers plenty of exercises to promote advertising awareness and celebrate actual, real-life feminine beauty. For boys, it might be particularly helpful for the father to have a talk with sons about how most models are unhealthy and are almost always airbrushed to look thinner and flawless. Boys can be encouraged to recognize that real feminine beauty and sex appeal has to do with the whole person—how a woman carries herself, how she interacts with others, and who she is as an individual.

It is critical that parents stay aware of the messages their children are being given. This awareness is a great tool in helping them to decipher fact from fiction, and to give them back their birthright: to feel comfortable in their bodies, and to eat until they are satisfied.

CHANGING THE PATTERN

PARENTS

❧ Buy some of the magazines marketed to teens. Educate yourself about their content so you can talk with your teen about the pros and cons of what's inside. Be willing to listen and learn together.

❧ Do what you can to counteract the negative messages being fed to your children, whether by reducing their exposure, or talking to them about advertising, or both.

❧ Spend a good amount of quality time with your teen. In particular, dads can have a very positive impact on their daughters' self-esteem.

❧ Encourage your teen to get involved in activities outside the home, and to have a variety of friends.

TEENS

❧ Educate yourself about the lies and misinformation the media is propagating. One excellent resource is Dove's Campaign for Real Beauty—visit the website at www. campaignforrealbeauty.com.

✎ Broaden your horizons: At your age, the best way to set yourself up for a bright future is to have several interests and a variety of friends.

✎ Ask yourself honestly how you feel about yourself after watching a lot of commercials, or looking at fashion magazines—which are mostly full of ads. Ask yourself whether it's healthy to feel that way, and whether you're going to let the marketing industry have that kind of power over you. Take charge of your own future.

Scenario 20

AN ISLAND UNTO HIMSELF

WHEN OVERWEIGHT TEENS

START TO WITHDRAW

Life is either a daring adventure or nothing.
—Helen Keller

Being overweight as an adult is difficult, but being overweight as a child or teenager can be devastating. Teens in particular long to be accepted by their peers, but in our thinness-obsessed society, this can be incredibly difficult for those who are overweight. As a result, many overweight teens feel ostracized by their peers due to teasing—or they may make a choice to seclude themselves from the outside world, where they just don't seem to fit in. This sense of separation is fertile ground for the development of various kinds of social problems. And in addition to feeling like outsiders, overweight children often develop an unbalanced relationship to food, particularly when well-intentioned parents attempt to restrict calories or otherwise control their eating.

In the following scenario, fourteen-year-old Charlie has been struggling with his weight his entire life and believes the only way he's going to have any control over what he wants to eat is to take matters into his own hands.

THE DAY DAD DECIDED TO GET A SECOND

job to supplement his teacher's salary was the day everything got better. Rick and Gina, my older brother and sister, are in college now, and a couple of months ago, they told Mom and Dad they're having a hard time getting by because of how expensive food and rent are. That's why it was decided that it was time for Dad to find a way to earn a little more money. He's now the track coach at the local high school, so he's always busy after school.

With Dad out of the picture, I don't have to eat all the fruits and vegetables he wanted me to snack on in the afternoons. I can finally eat what I want to eat, without worrying about being caught. I don't even have to be sneaky about eating the Twinkies, cookies, and candy I get on the way home, stuffing them in my backpack and hiding them under my bed.

I don't like having to be dishonest with Mom and Dad, but they'd be really upset if they found out. That's why I've been very clever about the whole thing. I want to make sure it's virtually impossible for them to ever discover any evidence, so I devised a fail-safe plan. Under my bed is a big green garbage bag. That's where all the wrappers and other garbage goes. It's also where I toss most of the fruits and vegetables that Dad sets out for me to eat after school—that's to make sure he thinks I'm eating them. Once a week, the day before the garbage man comes, and when Mom and Dad are still at work, I take the bag out and put it into the can. Just to be doubly sure that no one discovers the evidence, I make sure I stuff it under the rest of the garbage.

Now I am home-free. I love being home alone after school—having the house to myself. No more worrying about Dad walking in on me while I'm eating what I want to eat. I can play my video games full blast while I eat, because I don't have to worry about whether or not I can hear his footsteps coming down the hall.

I guess there's a downside to all my sneaking around. I have noticed that my pants are getting tighter, and that my favorite shirt doesn't button on the bottom anymore. It's kind of obvious that I'm still getting bigger, but maybe that's just the way I'm meant to be. Mom and Dad haven't said anything about it lately, anyway. I guess they've both been too preoccupied with financial stuff lately. They aren't even suspicious that I don't ask for dessert or after-dinner snacks anymore, even though I used to practically beg for them. The begging never worked anyway, so now I've taken matters into my own hands.

What do people expect from me? I have been on some sort of diet my entire life. I've always been chubby. I was even chubby as a baby. Mom told me that when I was two, the pediatrician told her she should limit how much I ate or else I would grow up to be fat. But it doesn't seem fair. Rick and Gina never have to worry about their weight. Why couldn't I have gotten some of their athletic genes? I'm so sick of being told what I can and cannot eat, especially when everyone else gets to eat whatever they want. For as long as I can remember, Mom has always made me a "special dinner" and even makes a point to dish it up, just for me. She said I should feel special, but having to eat something different from the rest of the family just makes me feel even worse, like there's something wrong with me. I want to make my own choices and eat what the rest of the family is eating. I hate feeling like everyone is watching every bite of food I put into my mouth.

The kids at school don't help the situation either. They make fun of me every chance they get. Walking between classes is a nightmare. Kids I don't even know make rude comments about me, calling me "lard butt" and "chunk boy." Gym class is the *worst.* I'm always the last to be chosen for any team, no matter what the sport. If any of those kids had any idea how much I rock on guitar, they'd probably stop making fun of me. Or maybe they wouldn't. I don't know. Maybe they'd just think I was a fat geek in the school jazz band. I guess you have to be an athlete to be popular. And that's never going to be me. Even if I wanted to play sports, I'd probably never be any good at them, or I'd just make a fool of myself. It would just give the kids at school one more reason to make fun of me.

Home is my refuge, the only place I can relax. I can play my favorite video games and munch on my favorite foods. Sometimes I get lost in the world of the game, forgetting who I am in this world and becoming a super hero, fighting my arch enemies and rescuing people in distress. In the game, I have the strength and agility to swing my body in any direction I want. I am in control. I enter those worlds, and I'm not sure how, but my food stash disappears. All I know is that I get to eat the food I like, and I finally feel calm.

POINTS TO PONDER

Charlie was a smart, imaginative, and musically talented boy. But since he felt that people were trying to control him everywhere he turned, he decided he had no choice but to take things into his own hands, developing a sort of "it's me against the world" mentality. He channeled his energy into developing intricate schemes, taking tremendous satisfaction in outsmarting others. He sought the safety and comfort of his room, where he could decide what and how much he ate. In his room, his imagination could run free in the fantasy world of his video games, where he was the hero, and no one would tease him about being fat.

When Charlie's parents took him, at the age of two, to the pediatrician and were told that they must limit his food intake or he would become a fat kid, they did what most parents would do: They followed the doctor's advice, believing completely that they were doing the right thing. But in reality, they were unwittingly setting Charlie up for a lifelong struggle with his weight. Unfortunately this happens all too often, because people believe that if a child is overweight, he eats too much, and in order to be thin, he must eat less. The fact is that most overweight kids eat no more than their normal-weight peers. Some do eat more, but that is more the exception than the rule. The reality is that some children will never be thin, but that doesn't mean they can't be healthy.

Even though they are making an informed choice to do so, parents who understand the importance of allowing overweight children to have control over their own eating habits may feel as if they are swimming upstream, because of the societal pressure they feel to have a normal-weight kid. After all, childhood obesity has become a hot topic in the media. There is increasing concern about what children are eating, and evidence that weight-related health problems—such as Type 2 diabetes and heart disease—are occurring at younger and younger ages.

However, parents must be careful about the message they are sending to their children. It is important to make sure that kids are not anxious about their bodies and the food they eat. Ellyn Satter, a nationally recognized nutrition expert and author of *Your Child's Weight: Helping Without Harming,* said that the key is to teach children to be "joyful and competent with eating."

That kind of lesson sets children up for a lifetime of healthy eating choices, and to be more accepting of their bodies.

Open communication between parents and teens begins in childhood and can help everyone get their needs met. Teenagers especially need to feel they can talk about their problems and express their feelings without having them taken over and solved by their parents. This is a delicate balance to achieve but a necessary step in empowering teens to trust in themselves. Teens need and deserve to feel that they have a voice in decisions that affect them.

Had Charlie shared with his parents how isolated he was feeling, perhaps they could have suggested that he get involved in activities that were more comfortable for him—activities that fostered his talents. A chess club would be a healthy way for him to channel his intelligence and love of strategy. Maybe if he had started his own band, he could have developed friendships with kids of similar interests.

It's not clear whether Charlie ever had an actual conversation with his parents about how much he hated having them control what he was allowed to eat; however, we did see that he practically begged for desserts and after-dinner snacks but was denied. It was probably difficult for Charlie to have a grounded conversation with his parents about this emotionally charged topic, especially since he would have been approaching it from a place of powerlessness—because when parents control their children's eating, a sense of powerlessness is often created. And from there, disordered eating and even a full-blown eating disorder may develop.

Instead of restricting his calories, Charlie's parents may have been able to get him help in a more productive way. A registered dietitian could have 1) helped Charlie develop a more positive relationship with food, 2) explained to the family how it would be best for Charlie to take charge of his own eating and exercise habits, and 3) emphasized staying active over counting calories. True, Charlie did not see himself as an athlete, but everyone can benefit from exercise, without having to excel or win awards. Charlie's father, who was a track coach, might have been able to develop an exercise routine with him—one they created together and could practice together—or helped him find a sport that he enjoyed. If Charlie didn't feel comfortable doing team sports, he might have enjoyed some individual activities, like biking or hiking. Learning a martial art would be an excellent way for Charlie to embody the hero he imagined himself to be in his video games. This kind of activity would help Charlie build self-esteem as well as strength and body confidence.

A positive experience in athletics—whether it be individual or team-related—can help prepare a young person to enter the bigger world with more self-assurance. Sports can also build teens' endurance and allow them to get in touch with their bodies in a way that has nothing to do with appearance. By learning how to work with others toward a common goal, and by developing new skills, teenagers begin to feel more competent. They learn to take risks: how to win and how to lose. They also learn how to put forth their best effort. They learn how to fail, recover, and survive intact.

Despite the claims of success they hear from the media—or even from a family doctor—parents should resist the temptation to put a child on a diet. Diets have been linked to a decrease in self-esteem that can last a lifetime. They can also interfere with the nutritional needs of a growing child and can create long-term health risks. In addition, diets teach children not to trust their bodies, and to disregard their own body's cues of hunger and fullness.

Also, it is particularly important that one child is not singled out to eat special foods, while the rest of the family eats something else. Not only will the child eventually rebel, but this can negatively impact family relationships. In that kind of environment, children learn to hoard food, eat secretively, and feel even worse about themselves. When the rest of the family eats the same foods as overweight children, the kids don't see eating healthfully as a punishment, and food does not become "the enemy."

In addition to serving everyone the same dishes, it's a good idea to make sure teens have regular access to snacks and treats— at school and at home—and that whenever possible these snacks be regular and planned, as opposed to just being a free-for-all, in which teens can graze all day without awareness.

Making family mealtime a pleasant experience, and trying to eat together as often as possible (three or more times a week) provides a wonderful opportunity for busy families to connect. If the dinner meal doesn't work, try breakfast or lunch. Establishing a minimum of thirty minutes per meal helps everyone eat more slowly and appreciate the meal—and each other. Eating slowly also helps us determine when we have eaten enough so that we can avoid overeating. Make sure the TV and laptops are nowhere around during mealtimes—these distract from our bodily cues of fullness and hunger, and impair good family communication.

People come in all shapes and sizes, and some people aren't genetically programmed to be thin. That's why it is highly important that large children be taught that their self-worth has nothing to do with their weight. With regular exercise, good communication, quality time as a family, and perhaps a few visits to a registered dietitian, overweight teens can learn to enjoy food and enjoy feeling good in their bodies.

CHANGING THE PATTERN

PARENTS

❧ Take the focus off scales and pounds, and instead promote healthy eating and lifestyle habits, including exercise. Exercising as a family is always a great thing.

❧ When it comes to food, treat your overweight child or children the same as other siblings. Provide healthy meals and snacks for everyone, and allow each child to determine how much he or she eats.

❧ Encourage your teen to get involved in meal planning and preparation, and put a little effort into making foods look attractive and appealing on the plate.

✺ Maximize opportunities for your child to get active. The longer a child has been sedentary, the harder it is to reverse the trend.

✺ Pay close attention to your child's individual interests, abilities, and personality, and try to devise ways—with his help—to channel them into activities that promote an active and social lifestyle.

TEENS

✺ Find something active that you enjoy doing. Make it fun!

✺ Be honest with yourself, and your loved ones, about any unhealthy eating habits you may be struggling with. All foods can be part of a healthy diet when eaten in moderation. Ask your family for help if you need support, so that you can enjoy the foods you like without worrying.

✺ Pursue interests that you enjoy. Not everyone is an athlete, and that is perfectly okay. Everyone has unique gifts and talents.

✺ Take responsibility for what you eat and how active you are.

Scenario 21

EVERYBODY ELSE'S GIRL

WHEN TEENS BECOME CARETAKERS

It is not a bad thing that children should occasionally, and politely, put parents in their place.

—Sidonie-Gabrielle Colette

Girls with eating disorders are often inclined to be caretakers and put other people's needs before their own. Sometimes a teen with this tendency takes excessive care of her own parents, especially when her parents' schedules are so busy that the children and housework aren't getting proper attention. Because she is focusing on what she can do to take care of a mother or father, the teen becomes disconnected from her own needs. This dynamic is fertile ground for the onset of an eating disorder, because the girl has no place to turn for her own nurturing. An empty vessel, she tries to fill herself up with high-calorie food to fill the void.

In the following scenario, sixteen-year-old Betsy is accustomed to anticipating her mother's every wish and puts aside activities and friends so that she can take care of her family's household chores.

"BETSY, CAN YOU GET DINNER STARTED TO-

night? I'm going to be late getting home from work. Sorry. It won't happen again, I promise."

I had heard these words before. More and more often, Mom was asking me to "start" dinner, which usually meant "make the whole meal." I love Mom, and I know her job as an attorney is really demanding. It's just that it's hard to put my homework aside and think about what to cook for dinner. It would have been nice to actually finish my homework, or to call my friend Carol. I knew it was too much to hope for Carol to call me. She knows I don't have much time to talk after school because I am always busy cooking dinner or putting in a load of wash before my mom comes home. Dad hates housework and leaves it up to "the women" to get the house chores done. I know what "the women" means—it means *me.* Who else is there to do it? It's days like today that I wish I had a brother or sister to share the load.

I know that Mom sometimes stops off at the gym on the way home to work out before she hits the front door. She's always in a better mood when she exercises, but when do *I* have a chance to exercise or do anything *I* want to do? Never.

Oh, well, I thought. *Why fight it?* I went downstairs, got some tuna out of the pantry and threw a casserole together. Just like the perfect little housewife. Argh! I was so mad. I knew I needed to find a way to tell Mom that this just wasn't fair. She didn't seem to be picking up on the hints I'd been trying to give her. Sometimes I slam the door hard when I'm mad, but she just says, "Careful, sweetie," and goes on with what she is doing. If I told her outright that something has to change, I know she'd apologize, but nothing would really change.

If I didn't already know she was a smart and successful attorney, I'd think she was totally clueless. She definitely acts clueless when it comes to knowing about what I think and feel. Aren't moms supposed to read between the lines and know what you are thinking? Not my mom. I wonder if she has any idea how much this affects my social life. Can she really be this selfish, or are kids supposed to do this much housework? One thing is for sure—my friends aren't chained to the stove and the washer and dryer like I am. But then my friends' moms aren't important downtown attorneys who can't exercise until after work. I guess I should be proud of her. But I get so angry about this.

I didn't know what to do, or who to talk to. I knew Dad wouldn't get it, and it's not the kind of thing you take to the school counselor. Mom had to be the one. But the thought of confronting her about it was so scary. After the casserole was in the oven, I sat down at the table to get some homework done. I heard my mother's car drive into the garage. *It's now or never*, I thought. *I have to work up the courage to do this.*

As my mom walked in the door and deposited her gym clothes in the laundry room, I tried to intercept her path. "Hey, Mom, do you have a minute?" I said. My heart was pounding. The last thing I wanted was to tick her off and make things worse.

"Sure, honey. Let me take a quick shower first and then I'll be right down."

"Mom, this can't wait. I'll lose my courage."

"Betsy, don't be so dramatic. You know I'm easy to talk to. What is it?" Mom walked to the kitchen, pulled a beer out of the refrigerator, and sat down at the table. "Mmmm. That casserole smells good, Betsy. Now what is it? Can't be that bad."

"Mom, I don't know how to tell you this. I've been trying to tell you in my own way for months—maybe years—and you are just not getting it."

"Betsy, are you having some problem at school, with your friends? What's the matter? I'm starting to get worried."

"Mom, I am sick and tired of fixing dinner every night and being in charge of the laundry. I feel like a mom myself, and

I'm too young to be strapped with all this housework. It just isn't fair to me." I was trying hard not to cry.

Mom frowned. "What is this, Betsy? You've never talked like this before."

"Mom, I am sixteen years old, and I want to do things after school with my friends or even do my homework. Can't you understand that? I am just a normal kid who wants to have some free time once in awhile." I couldn't help it; I was crying now and watching my mother's surprised face. This had to be the hardest thing I had ever done.

"Betsy, you're the one being unfair. You don't cook dinner *every* night. That is a huge exaggeration. And don't forget all the vacations we can take because I work so hard. If I try to get home earlier and have to cook dinner, that's all over, because I won't get my billables in. Think about that. You love going to the Caymans, don't you?"

She wasn't getting it, and I was feeling defeated already. Still, I kept on. "Mom, the Caymans don't mean anything if this is the price I have to pay. Can't you understand that? I don't mind helping you out once in awhile, but I don't have a life because of this. Just let me have a life, Mom. I'm going to lose all of my friends if I can never do anything with them."

She just shook her head and got up. "Betsy, I can't think about this anymore right now. I need to take a shower before that casserole is out and Dad gets home. Can you just throw together a salad real quick? I'll be right down, and we'll talk some more."

I couldn't believe it. I watched my mom get up and head toward the stairs. I sat there for a few minutes, wondering why it never worked to try to explain something important to my mom. I finally got up and found a package of salad mix in the refrigerator, threw it in a bowl, and cut up some tomatoes. I threw a piece of plastic wrap over the bowl, shoved the whole thing back into the fridge, and headed for my room. My job was done.

Casserole and salad didn't sound good to me at all. Dinner almost never sounds good anymore. But that's okay. I know how to feel better. I have a big bag of peanut M&M's hidden in my bottom dresser drawer. When I feel like this, I just pig out on candy until it's almost time to eat; then I throw it up to make room for dinner so I can put on a show of eating a decent meal with Mom and Dad. This started about a year ago and happens more and more often, usually on the nights I have to cook. Fortunately, my parents haven't caught on. I'd be really embarrassed, and besides, it's really comforting to do it. It's like my own private time, with my own private thoughts. Sometimes it feels like the only real freedom I have.

POINTS TO PONDER

Betsy was a teen who had been trained to take care of her mother. Because her mother worked hard and made a lot of money, she felt justified in burdening her daughter with taking care of the household chores. Betsy was troubled about how she should react to this, because even though it didn't seem fair, she loved her mother and didn't want to face a confrontation. Apparently, she had tried before to let her mom know how she needed more free time, but until now, she never came right out and stated her feelings. Being so direct and confrontational was a big step for Betsy, and yet her mom still could not handle what she was hearing. She got away from Betsy as soon as she could and headed for the shower, leaving Betsy to deal with her feelings by herself. Betsy turned to candy for comfort and to give herself the nurturing she needed, in the only way she knew how.

Girls with eating disorders are often caretakers, and have either been trained or have chosen to put their own needs aside in order to please the people that are important to them. Betsy was in touch with her anger, but many girls who are caretakers are not. A teen with this caretaking pattern has learned to focus on others, and often has a hidden resentment that sits underneath the helping behavior. In a family where parents are absent, too busy to listen, or preoccupied, it can seem fruitless to try to get their attention. Sometimes the caretaking behavior keeps escalating, because the teen thinks that if she just tries harder to please, her parents will finally notice what she needs and give her the attention she is missing. If the pattern goes on too long, she may give up and look elsewhere for a source of nurturing. In Betsy's case, it was chocolate.

Betsy's mother was so focused on her work that she couldn't see what her daughter was longing for. Schedules that are this packed have a way of blinding one to the needs of others. If Betsy's mother could have taken a few minutes to really hear her daughter, the result might have been a compromise about the housework and, more importantly, a better relationship with her daughter. With the kind of income her mother made, she could have hired someone to prepare meals and do housework so that Betsy could meet her social needs and feel heard.

Betsy's dad was mysteriously absent in this scenario. We might assume that he was also too busy to be part of the solution. We know that he believed that housework is only for women. Betsy didn't feel that it would accomplish anything to talk to him either, so she probably was not very close with him. Not having either parent available to hear one's feelings is an especially lonely situation.

Listening doesn't have to take a lot of time. It just takes focusing and caring. A few words like, "Betsy, I am so glad you shared what you feel. We'll figure out something different. I'm sorry that you have felt so burdened" could have turned the entire conversation in a healing direction. And Betsy may have felt heard enough by her mother that she didn't need the candy to try to soothe her feelings.

So few words would have been required to tip this situation and create a more open conversation with a very different outcome. If Betsy's mother could have attained a slightly different mindset about what it takes to truly listen and solve a problem, it could have made all the difference, and she could have given her daughter the understanding she needed so badly.

Parents who expect their children to take care of them are usually well intentioned and unaware of the burden this expectation places on their teens. At this age, teens are trying to develop their own identities. They need to have some responsibilities in the family but also the room to discover who they are, separate from their parents. When parents really grasp this need and communicate to their teens the desire to change the pattern, they create a context that allows their children to begin the healing process.

CHANGING THE PATTERN

PARENTS

❧ Remember that your children still need to be heard and appreciated, even when you are busy and providing for the family.

❧ Take the time to examine whether or not your daughter is a caretaker. It may not be in the area of chores. It could be a tendency to take care of your feelings, and be more of a counselor than a daughter. If this is happening, see what you can do to take the pressure off her by finding outside help for yourself.

❧ Examine your own values about how you spend your time and what is really important. If you are overworking, ask yourself what that is about, and whether you need some help to get in balance.

⊗ Remember: Parenting is probably the most important job we undertake, and it can be the most rewarding. It requires being in the moment with your children and noticing what they need.

TEENS

⊗ Ask yourself whether or not you feel as if you take excessive care of a parent or other adults—or even your friends—without getting the same in return. You have a right to have your own time and life as a teen.

⊗ Talk to your parents about situations in which you don't feel heard.

⊗ When expressing yourself, frame your message as an "I" message by not placing blame on your parents, but by sharing your "feeling" reactions to what is disturbing you. Include a request about what you would like from them instead.

⊗ Remember that food can never replace love. It is meant to be a source of nutrition. Rather than turning to food as a temporary solution, start a conversation that can bring you closer to the ones you love.

Scenario 22

A NEW KIND OF FAMILY

WHEN DIVORCE STRIKES A TEEN'S LIFE

*If you don't like something, change it; if you can't change it,
change the way you think about it.*

—Mary Engelbreit

Divorce is a time of grief and anxiety for everyone involved. But it takes a particularly hard toll on teenagers, who are already going through so many transitions of their own. On top of all of the hormonal and body changes teens go through, they are also learning the ropes of a new social environment and trying to seek the acceptance of their peers.

When parents divorce, teens may feel abandoned by one or both of their parents. This may lead them to question their own identities, or whether or not they are really loved. They may even blame themselves for the split. If both parents do not stay actively engaged with their teens, assuring them that they are loved unconditionally, the teens are vulnerable to developing an eating disorder as a way of coping with difficult emotions.

In the following scenario, thirteen-year-old Tiffany is devastated by her parents' divorce and struggles with the feelings and changes she is forced to deal with when her life is turned upside down.

FINALLY, CHRISTMAS VACATION IS HERE. I have been looking forward to this for so long. I can finally sleep in and just take it easy. My first semester of middle school was challenging, to say the least. So much has changed.

I'm slowly starting to get used to it, but I felt like my life was turned upside down when my parents got divorced. At first, I couldn't believe it was happening. *How could Dad just fall out of love with Mom?* I wondered. *How can love just go away like that?* It was really scary. I'd never even considered that Dad might stop loving either me or Mom before. So for a while—even though he swore it wasn't true—I thought Dad must have stopped loving me too. Now I understand that it's not so much that he doesn't love me enough to stay. It's just that he doesn't love Mom anymore—and now he loves his new wife and wants to be with *her* instead of us.

I guess that's a little better, but it's still pretty awful. It hurts, but we're all doing our best to heal from it—especially me and Mom. Dad, on the other hand, is as busy as ever and seems pretty happy with his new wife and the cosmopolitan life that he's living in his tiny apartment in the city. It seemed like it was all so easy for him, and both me and my mom were really angry about that. It wasn't fair. For the first few months, I had to listen to Mom crying and yelling at Dad for hours on the phone. Sometimes when this was all going on, I would just lose it and scream, "What about *me?* Do you guys even *care* about what happens to me?"

Dad was pretty much out of the picture most of the time, so Mom had to deal with *all* of my anger about the divorce, even though Dad should have had to deal with it too. But how was I supposed to express how I really felt when the only time I saw him was at restaurants for lunch, or at his new place, with his stupid new wife hanging around? I felt bad that Mom had to put up with all my yelling and screaming when I got home. She was dealing with enough as it was, trying to figure out a way for the two of us to survive.

After the divorce, we had to sell the house, and I was basically forced to move out of the only home I'd ever known. Luckily, Mom and I found a smaller house that wasn't too far away, so I could stay in the same school district and still go to the same school that all my friends are going to. But even though I'm with the same group of kids at school, nothing feels the same anymore. Mom had to go back to work to support us, and she's never home when I get home from school. I know it seems stupid, but that's a big deal for me. I always looked forward to coming home and telling Mom about my day. Now when she gets home she seems so tired and distracted—or so bent on going to the gym and working out—that it doesn't seem right to bother her with my stuff.

My dad is another story. He seems so wrapped up with his new wife that when he asks me to visit (which isn't very often), I feel like an outsider. They don't even have a room for me to sleep in, and I end up sleeping on the couch in the middle of their tiny apartment. Talk about feeling out of place! And on top of that, he's always so busy with work that a few times he even forgot to meet me for the lunch dates we scheduled—which were to make up for the weekends he wasn't able to have me over. He might as well not even bother, because when he forgets about me, it only makes me feel worse.

Everything is totally weird and sad now. Mom's doing her best to help me. She knows how hard this is for me, and she's put a lot of effort into making our new home really comfortable. She even let me decorate my room the way I wanted, helping me paint crazy stripes on the walls, and letting me pick out my own bedspread and accessories.

Sometimes it feels like me and her against the world—which is sad, but it also makes me love her even more. She really needs my love right now, too. I know she's not feeling too great about herself. Ever since the divorce, she's been asking me if she looks fat in her clothes. She's always looking in the mirror and making negative comments about her body. We go to the gym together all the time now, which is great, but I have to admit I miss the old days, when she and I used to watch funny movies and eat buttered popcorn. Now it's all about watching calories. She's even decided to become a vegetarian, and she's trying to pull me on board. "We don't need all that meat anymore, right?" she said. "There's no man around here anymore. And besides, it's fattening."

School is different too. There are so many new kids, new teachers, and new classrooms to get used to. Even though I see most of my friends every day, I don't actually have classes with most of them. My best friend, Molly, doesn't have any of the same classes as me, and when I pass her in the hallway these days, I see her talking to some girl I don't even know. I feel jealous, which I know is wrong, because I know that Molly and I will always be friends. But part of me is scared that I'm going to lose her too, and then what would I do?

There's something else that's really spooked me. I never really got any attention from boys before. I was always "the tall girl." But a couple months ago, I noticed some of the older boys eyeing me in the cafeteria. They were pretty cute too! So cute that I couldn't help blushing as I carried my tray over to my table of friends. All of a sudden it hit me: *Wow. Maybe Mom is right. Maybe I'd better start paying more attention to my looks and watching what I eat.* I tossed the sandwich and dessert I'd just bought into the trash and just ate my salad. And I decided to make a real commitment to run or go to the gym every day. After all, I don't want to be one of those high school girls without a boyfriend, do I? I definitely don't want to grow up and be alone. Mom seems so sad without Dad. Maybe if she'd paid more attention to her looks when she was with Dad, he never would have left her for his new wife.

These realizations were so shocking that it was easy to start the eating and exercise regimen I designed that night. Before, I'd never really thought about how I looked, but now I do all the time. Unfortunately, it's getting harder and harder for me to look in the mirror. Even though it was easy to diet at first, I've started to hate it. I find myself thinking about food all the time. I even have dreams about it! Finally, I couldn't handle it anymore and caved in. I started stopping at the grocery store on the way home and buying a bag of all my old favorite munchies. All the forbidden ones, all the foods I hadn't been allowing myself to eat. Then when I get home I go straight to my room, lock the door, and have a feast. When I'm done, I make sure to hide all the evidence. I'd be mortified if Mom saw that I was pigging out like this.

I've gained back all the weight I lost, plus an annoying five more pounds. I wish I had more self-control! But I really don't care. The good news is I don't feel so anxious and depressed anymore. It seemed like when I was so focused on my body and what the boys at school thought of me, I was a total mess. I'm not interested in them or what they think anyway, because you can't really trust them. Now I can just relax. Besides, eating gives me something to do when I get home from school. The house doesn't feel so big and empty anymore. I've got my food to keep me company. It's always there for me.

POINTS TO PONDER

Tiffany's unhealthy relationship with food—bingeing, and then trying to go back to restricting to make up for it—stemmed in part from the fact that she reached an age where boys were suddenly interesting. Once this interest manifested, the messages that she'd been getting from her parents—both subtle and overt—began to kick in. From her mother, she was getting the underlying message that a skinny woman is more lovable than one who's not. From her father, she may have been getting a similar message—especially if his new wife was skinnier than her mom. Even without such messages from parents, teen girls in Tiffany's position can interpret this particular kind of divorce situation as "Love is fickle, and one must be captivating to hold a man's interest." That's a lot of pressure on a young girl.

Tiffany's initial response to her father leaving—"Don't you love me anymore?"—is extremely common. Even though she was eventually convinced that it wasn't true, her understanding of the nature of love was profoundly rocked by the divorce. This showed in her fearful reaction to seeing her best friend talking to another girl at school. As a result of the divorce, Tiffany suddenly realized that the people she loved most might leave her. This feeling—the fear of abandonment—can show up later in life, creating problems in adult relationships.

Tiffany's mother was a real trooper and was doing the best she could. Forced to start from scratch—to get a new house, and to go back to work to support herself and her daughter—was challenging enough. But on top of all that, she was also struggling with her own self-worth and body image. Perhaps as a coping mechanism, she turned to focusing on her body and her weight to avoid the more painful emotions she was experiencing.

Tiffany's father was totally absorbed in his new relationship and didn't make enough time for her. Although he may have been telling her that he loved her, and reassuring her that would never change, his behavior, intentional or not, sent a different message: "I love you, but you are not one of my top priorities."

Divorce is painful for all involved, but parents must take responsibility to ensure that their children's needs are met. Adolescents can feel betrayed by divorce and need reassurance that parents will provide some stability. Talking to them about their feelings and having individual time with them is essential.

Some teens may benefit from family or individual counseling. Things might have gone differently had Tiffany had a safe place—such as a therapist's office—to express all of her newfound worries, fears, anger, and sadness. As she stated herself, it wasn't really possible for Tiffany to communicate with her father about any of her concerns, because when they met, it was either in a public place or at his apartment, when his new wife—a stranger—was present. And although she and her mother had a wonderful, loving relationship, it's clear that Tiffany felt that her mom was struggling, and therefore should not be worried by Tiffany's concerns. In fact, she was probably worried that many of her feelings and her questions—such as "Is Mom sad and lonely because she needs to lose weight?" or "Why does love just go away?"—might cause more pain for her mother. By talking with a trusted adult who is unconnected with the situation, Tiffany might have been able to understand and correct some of these harmful ideas.

As a result of her newfound interest in boys, and her fear that being overweight means not being loved or being lonely, Tiffany attempted to control her food and her body by diet and exercise. Dieting at any age is not productive, but for a teen—who needs plenty of calories in order to grow—dieting is not just unproductive, it's harmful. It's even harder for a growing teen to control her appetite, so it's not surprising that Tiffany's attempt at dieting resulted in binge eating.

Binge eating usually occurs as a result of unsuccessful and repeated attempts to lose weight. However, Tiffany's case was different: She was probably turning to food as a comfort—a reaction to her painful struggles with her parents' divorce, as well as a new situation at school that she didn't know how to deal with. The secrecy and shame she experienced typifies the repulsion binge eaters feel about their own behavior, yet they seem unable to stop. Binge eaters suffer the same out-of-control eating experienced by people with bulimia, but they do not vomit or purge. The binge eater will generally consume large amounts of food quickly—almost without thinking, and most often, when they are not even hungry.

Tiffany, "the tall girl," was probably more physically mature than most of her peers. All of a sudden she was being noticed, and not just by boys her age, but by older boys. This was something that came to her as a shock, and she didn't know how to react to it. It was apparently and understandably a source of anxiety for her. In general, sexual anxieties can promote dieting—and, in turn, binge eating—as a way of coping with uncomfortable emotions. In addition, studies have shown that fast-maturing girls are at increased risk for eating disorders. Going through puberty happens at different times for each teenager, which can pose additional stress on the adolescent if she is not measuring up to the cultural ideal, or is ahead of the curve.

All parents should be sure to educate themselves about the normal stages of growth and development that their children are experiencing. Even without divorce, parents need all the information and preparation they can get about what lies ahead for them and their teens. By being aware and in tune, parents can foster better communication with teens during these critical times, when they want more autonomy but are also more easily influenced by their peers.

It is this communication that can make all the difference in the world. Parents and teens alike will be struggling with feelings of sadness and loneliness over the breakup of the family. But when both parents stay actively engaged with their children in order to assure them that they are loved unconditionally, true healing can begin.

CHANGING THE PATTERN

PARENTS

❧ Encourage your teen to get into counseling if she has experienced a trauma in their lives, such as a divorce or loss of a close friend or relative. This allows her to express difficult feelings in a safe environment.

❧ Never encourage your teen to diet. Instead, emphasize eating well and regular physical activity.

❧ If you're going through a divorce, make sure your teen has a safe place in an encouraging atmosphere to openly express to each parent her concerns. Encourage her to talk about the tough stuff.

TEENS

❧ Talk to your parents about what's going on in your life—even the stuff that is hard to talk about.

❧ Never deny how you feel. Your feelings are an important part of who you are. If you think you're not able to express them fully, suggest to a parent that you might be helped by a therapist.

❧ Avoid dieting. Find nonfood ways to de-stress (take a nap, listen to music, etc.).

❧ Try to get your proper rest during times of stress. Being well rested helps you better deal with difficult situations and feelings.

SUPPLEMENTARY READING:

FOR PARENTS

Growing Up with Divorce: Helping Your Child Avoid Immediate and Later Emotional Problems, by Neil Kalter

Scenario 23

UPROOTED

WHEN A TEEN IS
THE NEW KID IN TOWN

There are two lasting bequests we can give our children: One is roots, the other is wings.

—Hodding Carter Jr.

Sooner or later, many if not most families face the prospect of moving. As stressful and disruptive as moving can be on parents, it can be even more traumatic for their teenagers. Because they're in the process of developing their own identity, something like a major move—where they are leaving behind their tried-and-true social groups—can totally disrupt how they define themselves. To start a new school and gain a peer group's acceptance can be a daunting task, even for the most self-assured teen. As a survival strategy, a vulnerable teen may develop an eating disorder, thinking that if she is just thin enough, she will eventually be accepted into the desired social group.

In the following scenario, fifteen-year-old Gretchen has spent all of her life in Germany, but she suddenly finds out that her family is being relocated to the United States.

I WAS JUST PUTTING THE FINAL TOUCHES ON

the birthday cake that my *oma* and I baked for Becky's seventh birthday when Mom burst through the kitchen door in tears.

"Your father just found out he's being transferred to a military base in the United States," she said. *Oma* and I were stunned into silence.

Finally, I asked the question I was terrified to ask: "Do we have to go with him?" After all, Dad went on lots of temporary assignments that we didn't join him on. Maybe, hopefully, this would be one of those.

But Mom shook her head. "It's a four-year tour, so I'm sure we will."

I had to fight back the tears that were suddenly brimming in my eyes. "I can't leave my friends, especially not now, when I'm just about to start secondary school!"

Mom sighed. "Oh, Gretchen, I'm so sorry, I shouldn't have said anything yet. Especially not now, when we are having Becky's birthday party this afternoon." She put her arm around my shoulder, giving me a hug. "I was so upset myself after your dad called. I didn't even think before bursting in here. That's not fair to you. I hope you'll forgive me."

I couldn't help it anymore, and the tears started falling down my face. She wiped them away and kissed my cheek, saying, "I promise we will talk when Dad gets home tonight. I shouldn't have spoiled this special time for you and your grandmother. I know how much you two enjoy baking together." She stood up and looked at our creation. "Wow! Look at the cake you made for Becky! It's beautiful. She's going to be thrilled!"

I didn't say anything in response. I couldn't. Mom got quiet again and said, "Can we please not say any more about this right now and try to enjoy the party? Dad will tell us more about this when he gets home. Then we can figure out what's best—as a family, okay?"

I reluctantly agreed. And despite the overwhelming sadness we all felt, Mom, *Oma*, and I put on our best party faces and tried to enjoy watching Becky and her friends play the games we planned for them. When we brought in the birthday cake, twinkling with candles, Becky's eyes lit up. It was great, but there was also a dark cloud hanging over us.

My mom and dad met when Dad was stationed in Germany, so my sister and I have lived there all of our lives. Of course we visited Dad's side of the family in America a few times, and we love them, but we grew up with Mom's family. Even though I loved visiting Dad's family and seeing the United States, I never imagined myself living there. Four years away from my friends, my grandparents, and my cousins seemed like forever.

When we sat down that evening, Dad was all smiles. He couldn't wait to get back to the States. There were so many things he wanted me and Becky to see and experience, and he was anxious to show off his "lovely German family," as he called us. Besides, he had been away from his own family and country for fifteen years.

When he saw that I was far from excited, he turned to me, gave me a big hug, and said, "You know how much you and I enjoy watching American football together? Well, now we can go to some real games! What do you think?" He was so excited.

I was still sad, but Dad's enthusiasm was infectious. Maybe it would be okay. After all, we all had each other.

But then another thought hit me. "What about *Oma?*" I asked. "We can't leave her behind." As soon as it came out of my mouth I stopped. I don't know what I was thinking— of course she couldn't come. She'd have to leave *Opa,* her friends, and her wonderful home. We would never expect her to do that. Mom reached over and gave me a hug—she knew I was seriously bummed.

Then I looked over at Becky and saw how excited she was, and that even Mom was smiling. So I figured I could survive. We'd been through tough times before, like when Dad was deployed to Iraq. Times like that proved that, together, we could make anything work.

We decided that Mom and Dad would take a special trip to the new duty station in Texas to find housing. Then we would all leave Germany during the summer, so there would be plenty of time to adjust to our new surroundings before school started. Mom and Dad agreed to look for off-base housing so that we girls would have an opportunity to experience what living in America was really like. Mom and Dad suggested that I get involved in a sport or some other activity at my new school right away. That way, I'd meet friends quickly, and I'd feel more comfortable.

Not long after we moved to Texas, I found the activity I wanted to do: cheerleading! I saw the poster that announced the one-week summer training for tryouts. I'd have to learn a routine and perform it by myself in front of last year's squad. Even though I felt like an outsider, I thought my experience as a dancer would give me an advantage the other girls didn't have. And how great would it be for Dad to go to the high school football games and see me on the field, cheerleading!

I was delighted when I found out that I made the squad— well, I *kind of* made it. I was selected as an alternate, but I still got to go to cheerleading camp with the rest of the girls. Even though I had years of dance experience, during my training before the tryouts, I saw right away that cheerleading and dancing are pretty different, and I still had a lot to learn, so it was pretty amazing that I still got picked to be an alternate. I thought cheerleading camp would be the perfect way to make friends and get close to some girls before school started. Everything seemed like it was not only going to be fine, but great.

The campground was a beautiful place on a lake not too far from town. And the coaches were great. They introduced me to the other cheerleaders and made me feel very welcome. But the other cheerleaders were not friendly to me at all—at least not in private. In front of the coaches, they were all smiles with me, but when we were sent to our cabins to change for dinner, they completely ignored me, answering my questions and comments with stony silence. I was totally confused and wondered what I did wrong.

Then, the worst thing happened. One night I overheard two of the girls in my cabin talking about me, calling me "that big fat German girl." They were complaining about me, saying I spoiled their plans to have only their best friends on the squad. After that, I got pretty quiet and didn't try too hard to talk to the other girls. I just trained, but I didn't even try my best. I didn't want to do too well. I felt like the better I did, the more they would hate me. But I also felt like if I didn't do well, I might get kicked off the squad. And then where would I be? I'd start school without any friends, and people would probably make fun of me for getting kicked off. Plus, I think Dad would be really disappointed. He was so excited about going to the football games and seeing me cheer.

At dinner, I'd just sit in silence and listen to the other girls talk. The topic of discussion was always the same: how they looked, and dieting. They even complained to the camp cook that there were no fat-free options on the menu.

I was devastated by how cheerleading camp turned out. I just wanted to make friends. I'd never heard anyone call me fat in Germany. I'd always been proud of my strong, muscular build. I never worried about what I ate before, or paid any attention to all this low-fat and fat-free stuff that seemed to be so important to these American girls. Me and my friends in Germany never worried about what we ate. But I was determined to find a way to fit in. *Maybe if I lost some weight, those girls might see me differently,* I thought. So I decided to do some research when I got home.

Mom and Dad were dying to hear all about camp when I got home. Of course, I couldn't tell them what really happened. They would feel so bad, and would maybe even feel guilty for sending me there. I knew my parents were counting on me to make the most of this new adventure. I didn't want to disappoint them, and I knew I could make this work—somehow.

So when they asked me about camp, I just said, "It was fun, but a lot of work." I focused on telling them about all the moves and routines I learned and avoided talking about the girls. But of course they asked about that too.

"Did you meet any nice girls?" asked Mom.

I wanted to say "No, but I met a whole lot of mean ones." Instead I said, "Of course, I met lots of girls. We were in training all week long together!" I tried to keep the conversation quick, and as soon as I could, I went to my room and turned on my computer. In less than five minutes, I found several different websites that had plenty of information on losing weight and dieting. I tried to focus on ways to lose weight quickly. Lucky for me, there seemed to be plenty of really good strategies.

I admit it: I hate that I have to skip lunch at school and give up so many of the foods I love to eat. I feel hungry almost all the time, and I am constantly thinking about food. But regardless of the sacrifice, I am determined to lose weight and fit in with the other girls.

Normally I would be worried that my parents would notice my dieting and try to stop me. But luckily, they are both caught up in all the challenges they're facing because of the relocation. It's pretty easy to pretend to eat dinner. I've become very good at moving the food around on my plate so that it looks as if I've eaten more than just a few bites (this was one of the tips I learned on the Internet). I also read about another brilliant strategy for distracting parents from how much I'm eating and not eating. It's so simple, but so effective! I just offer to clear the table and do the dishes every night. The more helpful I am, the more they focus on that. So far, they haven't suspected a thing; they are just happy that I'm so helpful. Another thing I do is put on lots of layers; this helps hide the fact that I'm getting skinnier.

But I have to be more careful. Just the other morning, Mom said, "Isn't it too hot outside to be wearing a hoodie to school?"

But I was quick on my feet: "The air conditioning at school makes it really cold," I said.

"Oh, that makes sense, I guess," she said.

Phew. It felt a little gross to be lying to Mom like that. But it was partially true! Lately I have been feeling cold for some reason. So it wasn't really a lie. It was a perfect thing to say, though. Now I can start wearing sweaters and jackets all the time, and Mom will think she knows why.

Even though I got over that hurdle, there are other obstacles to deal with. Just the other day, Mom said, "Hey, Gretch, are you sure you are doing okay? We haven't had a chance to spend much time together recently, and I really miss that. You seem so quiet and preoccupied. How about you and I bake one of your wonderful cakes for dinner this weekend? You used to love doing that with *Oma*."

My reaction was surprising to her. "Mom, do you realize how fattening those cakes are, and how bad they are for you? No way!" I said.

Right away, I knew the look on her face spelled trouble. So I said I had to go to practice and got out the door as quickly as I could.

I just really hate living in America. I miss my friends back home. If I'd stayed in Germany, we'd all be having so much fun in secondary school together right now. And I especially miss my *oma*. I always felt like I could talk to her about anything, and we used to have so much fun laughing and baking in her wonderful old kitchen.

But I'm stuck here. That's just the way it is. So I have to keep going with this weight-loss regimen. I'm actually really proud of how successful I've been. The other cheerleaders haven't really noticed, and they haven't lightened up on me yet either. They're still ignoring me and are totally caught up in their own little group of friends. But you know what? The more weight I lose, the less I care.

POINTS TO PONDER

Gretchen's story illustrates the fact that no family is immune to eating disorders. No matter what their family situation is, all teenagers have a desire to fit in, to be accepted by their friends and peers—and many are willing to go to extremes to accomplish this. Many of the scenarios in this book illustrate how a lack of communication and family togetherness can contribute to the development of an eating disorder. But in this scenario, we see that even a teen from a very close-knit, communicative family can be vulnerable.

When families are confronted with a major change, such as a big move, both parents and kids become busy with their own challenges and may not communicate as effectively as usual. In this scenario, however, Gretchen and her parents had a good relationship and were generally able to discuss and resolve difficult issues as a family. Perhaps because she didn't want to worry her parents, Gretchen tried to deal with her demoralizing experience at cheerleading camp all by herself, instead of consulting with her mom and dad. She went to the Internet for information and found some very dangerous websites that actually promoted eating-disordered behavior. This left her parents out of the loop and unable to support her, which in turn allowed the eating-disordered behavior to become more entrenched. Although her reason for losing weight was to connect with her peers, she ended up feeling more isolated from them, and more disconnected from her feelings and her family.

If Gretchen admitted to her parents that she was having trouble making friends, and that the other cheerleaders were avoiding her, they might have been able to help her see that being on the cheerleading squad wasn't the best thing for her. Her father might have been able to explain that he didn't want her to be a cheerleader if that meant she was being mistreated, and could have told her that he would rather have her with him in the stands, cheering on the team from there. As a family, they could have found another activity for Gretchen to take part in—one where she could meet friendly kids and feel accepted.

Major transitions can be very difficult and traumatic for a teenager, whether it's a move to a new school, starting college, divorce, a death in the family, or some other life-changing event. In addition to the stress of leaving her friends and much of her family behind in Germany, and the worries about having to fit in at a new school, Gretchen had another major difficulty to deal with: understanding a new, foreign culture that glorifies thinness and often rejects diversity. This is a challenge that she needed help with—help from a loving and trusted adult.

Because teenagers are experiencing so many physical and emotional changes anyway, parents can be blindsided by the discovery of an eating disorder. It's typical for teens to become more self-absorbed, more rebellious, and less communicative as they begin to separate from their parents and establish their own identities. So it is usually difficult to distinguish normal adolescent behavior from what might be the beginning of an eating disorder.

Even conscientious parents can miss the very subtle signs of an eating disorder. Early detection can be improved by being alert to sustained changes in a teen's eating habits, not the occasional quirks that are part of growing up. For example, many teenagers go on diets to lose weight, but the diet is generally short-lived. It is when the diet is prolonged and the teen's preoccupation with body appearance and weight intensifies that it becomes cause for concern. Making frequent excuses not to eat with the family, playing with but not eating food, and making trips to the bathroom after meals are a just a few of the behaviors teens may exhibit. Social warning signs include withdrawal or isolation, and decreased interest in friends or hobbies. Physical symptoms include weight loss, which may be accompanied by teens' wearing layered clothing—to hide the evidence or just to stay warm, as people with anorexia are often cold.

During a big move or any other major transition, it is particularly important for parents to let teens know they *want* to hear about their concerns, and that they respect them. Also, by involving teens in big decision-making processes, parents can assure them that their best interests are being kept in mind. When dealing with a big move, all family members should set realistic expectations. Throughout the first year—and beyond, if necessary—parents would do well to check in frequently with teens to see how they are transitioning. Family meals and meetings are excellent arenas in which to make that happen.

A big move can present many challenges, but great growth and bonding can also come from this kind of change. Your family may grow closer—and you may learn more about one another— as you go through this new adventure together.

CHANGING THE PATTERN

PARENTS

≈ If your family is going through a major transition, make sure to ask lots of questions, such as "How can I help you through this?" and "What do you need from me?"

≈ Spend one-on-one time with your teen. Be curious and alert to your teen's motivations, fears, and insecurities.

≈ Educate yourself about the early warning signs of an eating disorder. Early intervention is more likely to result in recovery.

⮫ Make a point to meet the kids your teen is hanging out with. Invite them over to the house so you can get to know them and see how your teen interacts with them.

TEENS

⮫ Ask your parents for help when difficult situations arise. You don't have to go it alone.

⮫ If you're being teased at school or feel excluded, let your parents know. They can support you and suggest ways to remedy the situation.

⮫ Look for friends who have similar interests and enjoy doing things you enjoy. Be willing to try something else if what you are doing isn't working out.

⮫ Free yourself from expectations about how you "should" look. Who you are as a person is always more important than what you look like.

Scenario 24

TWO WORLDS COLLIDE

WHEN A TEEN STRUGGLES
WITH BICULTURAL ISSUES

Do I contradict myself?
Very well then I contradict myself.
(I am large, I contain multitudes.)
—Walt Whitman

As the world shrinks, growing up in two cultures becomes an increasingly common experience for American children. When these children reach their teen years, the experience can become a struggle to try to fit in—both with the culture of their heritage and with the dominant culture in which they are living.

The teen years are a time to find one's place among peers and still feel grounded in family. Acceptance is important in both contexts. If this struggle seems impossible to resolve, a teen may develop symptoms of depression. When the difference revolves around cultural expectations of beauty and body image, the teen is susceptible to an eating disorder. If her family's orientation is less focused on thinness, she fears failure if she is not successful at restricting food but also fears rejection if she seems to turn her back on her family's image of beauty—an image that does not involve unhealthy thinness. Struggling with what feels like a no-win situation, she can feel defeated and develop symptoms that need attention from parents and professionals.

In the following scenario, fifteen-year-old Jennifer tries to explain to her mother how difficult this dilemma is for her, and longs for her mother's understanding.

"MOM, YOU JUST DON'T UNDERSTAND! WHY

can't you listen?" I turned on my heels and left the kitchen. I was so frustrated, because Mom just can't seem to get it through her head how much I *hate* my body.

I felt guilty about being so angry with Mom, though. I knew it was hard for her to understand a lot of things about my life. Even though she left San Blas with my grandparents when she was my age, and moved to the United States, settling in a neighborhood that didn't have any Mexican Americans, she never really tried to blend in here. She just focused on her family life. She doesn't really know what America is like outside her own little world. So I know why she has trouble empathizing, but I want so much for her to understand. Other than this big problem, she and I have a wonderful relationship. She is so loving, and she always tells me I'm pretty and curvaceous—but I don't feel curvaceous, I feel fat. My body is different from the bodies of most of my friends—who are all on a diet—and Mom just doesn't understand why that's even a problem for me!

The whole conversation started when I was so upset and confused that I couldn't even think anymore. I decided, once again, to tell my mom about why I've been feeling so crazy lately. I hoped that this time she would get it.

I found Mom in the kitchen, cooking dinner. She looked busy, but I hoped she would take time to listen. I flopped down at the table and opened a diet soda. "Mom, I need to talk to you," I said.

"Let me just stick these enchiladas in the oven, and I can rest for a minute," she said. I looked with longing as the pan of enchiladas went into the oven. I've always loved Mom's homemade enchiladas—the same recipe my grandmother used. The aroma reminds me of our family dinners in Mexico and the lively conversations around the table.

I was determined not to eat the enchiladas at dinner, though. The amount of fat they contained was huge. Enchiladas were definitely not on my list of acceptable foods. I drank my soda and strengthened my resolve. If I picked at the enchilada and pushed it around the plate, maybe my mother wouldn't notice.

After taking a couple of minutes to clean up, Mom sat down at the table and looked at me intently. "What's on your mind, Jen? You look troubled."

"Mom, this is hard to talk about," I said, trying not to cry. "I'm worried about so many things. I don't know whether you will understand or not." I was torn between telling her the truth and deciding at the last minute to make something up so she wouldn't worry. I struggled for composure but decided I had nothing to lose by telling her how afraid I was of food, and how much I hated my body.

"Mom, I just can't eat your enchiladas right now, or anything that is not on my safe list. If I don't cut calories, I will never be thin like my friends. They're always talking about safe foods, like yogurt and salads, when they come over here. But that's not how our family eats. You know how much I love your enchiladas, but they're so high in fat. Please don't take it personally, Mom." I wiped my tears on my sleeve and looked down at the table. I didn't want to look at my mother's disappointed expression and see that I had hurt her feelings.

But I didn't hurt her feelings, because she didn't even seem to take me seriously. "*M'hija,* you're being ridiculous," she said. "What are you talking about, 'safe foods'? Are you saying my enchiladas are dangerous? Who told you about that? Those girls you bring over here are too skinny, you know that. Uncle Tony even says so. Why would you want to be all bones like them? That's not pretty. You're so beautiful, Jen, everyone thinks so! Why can't you see that? Come on over here, taste my *mole*. Tell me it's not safe."

And that's when I lost my temper with her and stormed out.

It's true: Not just Uncle Tony, but all of my aunts and uncles tell me that I'm beautiful and that my friends are too thin. But they're just saying that. And the guys in my class obviously don't think so. I haven't been asked out once! If it keeps up like this, I'm not going to have a date for homecoming or junior prom. Thoughts like this make me miserable, and unfortunately, I'm having thoughts like this all the time now. It makes me feel like I hate myself, and sometimes I wish I could just go to sleep and never wake up. I know feelings like that aren't healthy, but I can't tell anyone about them. My family would be terrified if they found out.

Sometimes I wish my family would all move back to Mexico, or at least to a part of town where there are more Mexican Americans. That way, there'd be more girls like me, and I wouldn't feel so alone. I would miss Sarah and Amy, of course, but lately I can't even enjoy their company because I feel so depressed. Lately I've even been missing school—saying I'm sick—because I can't stand to face other people when I'm this down. Besides, the classes are all so pointless and boring, and my grades aren't even really suffering yet because of it.

So every once in a while, I take a deep breath and try to explain to Mom how I don't feel like I belong anywhere. But her reaction is always confused, and it doesn't seem like she believes me. "That's ridiculous, Jennifer," she always says. "When are you going to accept yourself exactly the way you are? You shouldn't feel that way. You're young; you should be happy! You look perfectly fine." Even though it's her best way of trying to make me feel better, it hurts when she reacts like that, and I end up feeling more alone than ever. *If I'm being ridiculous,* I think, *why am I so worried? What is wrong with me?*

Every summer, we all go to Mexico for two weeks to visit my Dad's side of the family. I love those trips, but they're confusing too. All my cousins hug me and tell me how great I look. We all gather around my grandparents' huge mesquite table and enjoy homemade tacos and rice that just don't taste the same as they do in California. My grandmother is an excellent cook, and no one worries about how much they're eating. During those meals, when the family is together again, sharing stories and laughter, I forget my insecurities. I feel embraced by the love and acceptance of my relatives. I feel perfectly accepting of my body, and I know for certain that no one there thinks I look too fat. My cousins' friends are even attracted to me and compete with each other to see who gets to take me to the beach or the market!

On the plane ride home, I always feel so strong and confident that I'm sure I can keep up my self-esteem and the positive feelings about my body. But it doesn't last long at all. As soon as I start walking to the baggage claim, I feel my mood drop and my stomach sink when I see the other girls in the airport. Most of them have skinny legs and sharp collar bones and look great in those skimpy summer shorts. Sure, not all the girls look like that, but it's as if the skinny girls are the only ones I see. I start wishing again, wishing so much that I looked like them. But I know that's impossible, and I start to feel helpless almost immediately. All of those great feelings that comforted me during the last two weeks disappear in an instant, and I find myself wondering, *How can I feel so differently about myself in two different places?*

I don't know what to do. I know my mom is trying to be reassuring, but she doesn't understand how important it is to fit in where we live. Dad is even harder to talk to—he travels every week on business, and on weekends, he needs to catch up on sleep and help Mom with bills and chores. Besides, he wouldn't know what to say even if I did tell him I hate my body. He loves a curvaceous Latina look and even teases me sometimes about eating too little. No one understands my dilemma.

My friends here at home are all super thin and dieting constantly, but my friends and cousins in Mexico love eating and couldn't care less about changing their bodies. I don't think they even understand the concept of dieting in San Blas! I feel so stuck. If I'm going to be popular, I have to lose weight. But even if I diet and I succeed in losing weight, my family will think I'm too skinny and say I'm trying to be like a *gringa*. If I go to San Blas next summer as a skinny girl who refuses to eat all that fattening food that my grandmother makes, everyone will see me as an outsider—or they'll bother me until I start acting like one of them again.

I just don't know how I can exist in two worlds at once. It's impossible!

POINTS TO PONDER

Body image is the most important component of an adolescent girl's self-esteem, especially in European American culture. Jennifer was struggling with extreme body dissatisfaction that could have easily led to an eating disorder if her concerns continued to get dismissed and she didn't receive professional help. She was also caught between two cultures that tend to view body shape and size in different ways. Latino standards of beauty are quite different from European American standards. Jennifer felt normal and accepted in Mexico but insecure in California. Her first-generation mother wasn't as acculturated as Jennifer and had difficulty understanding her daughter's dilemma, even though she tried to be reassuring.

Jennifer also showed classic symptoms of depression—a depressed mood, no pleasure in previously enjoyed activities, low self-esteem, and suicidal thoughts. It is not unusual for a teen with body-image dissatisfaction to be depressed, but in Jennifer's situation, it is not clear which came first. Was she depressed first, which contributed to her negative body image, or was the depression just one aspect of her doubts about her body? In any case, she was trying to be acceptable in two cultures with varying ideas about the importance of thinness, and this difference contributed to her unhappiness.

Her dilemma was intensified by the fact that she didn't know how to get help. She didn't think her mother would ever take her situation seriously enough to listen; instead of hearing her very real concerns, Jennifer's mother, with the best intentions, tried to convince her that she was overreacting. The cultural differences made it hard for Jennifer's mother to see the seriousness of Jennifer's concerns. She tried to be reassuring, but Jennifer felt, instead, that her feelings were being ignored. Regardless of culture, it is important for parents to tune in to the feelings behind their teen's concerns and start a conversation that reveals more information, instead of trying to dissuade the teen from worrying.

Because of the cultural difference, Jennifer's mother was particularly blind to the situation. And because Jennifer's worries were dismissed, the conversation came to a dead end. Thus, Jennifer's mother was not able to find out that her daughter needed help, and that she was having suicidal thoughts. Even if her mother did begin to see the seriousness of the situation, we wonder whether the cultural difference might have impeded her mother from getting professional help. It may have been that her mother had a cultural tendency to rely on strong family support as a sufficient answer to difficulties and would have closed her mind to sending Jennifer to a mental health professional, or to the use of antidepressants if the doctor made that recommendation.

It is difficult but important for parents to move beyond their own experience and hear their teens' fears and despair. With her mother's understanding, Jennifer would have been able to air her feelings and develop hope that she could resolve her unhappiness. Since she was suffering from a major depression, as well as the onset of an eating disorder, she needed professional help *and* her mother's support. In the best case, Jennifer's mother would have been open to locating a psychologist, social worker, or counselor trained in treating both depression and body-image concerns, and she would also have been willing to seek medical consultation. If Jennifer's worries were never taken seriously, she may have developed a full-blown eating disorder and experienced a worsening of her suicidal thoughts.

Ideally, a teen like Jennifer would do best with a bicultural therapist, someone who lives in the dominant American culture but also understands her family background. But this decision would depend on the teen's own degree of acculturation, and ultimately, she needs to work with whomever she feels most comfortable. Group therapy with other Latinas would have offered Jennifer interaction with other females like her—girls and women who could have related to her need to belong and to her feelings of being caught between two cultures. Family therapy could have helped Jennifer and her parents come to an understanding of their mutual needs. It could have helped her parents support her journey out of her depression and toward greater acceptance of her body. This type of therapy is often one in which Latinos feel the most comfortable, as traditional Latino culture is centered around the family.

Jennifer's struggle to fit in is not unique. It is every teen's struggle, regardless of culture, and when a teen is straddling the expectations of two cultures with differing body image expectations, the problem can seem overwhelming. The eating disorder may indicate a desperate attempt to be accepted, and the depression can be a serious symptom that the teen is feeling hopeless about resolving the struggle. Parents and other family members should try to understand this need to fit in and should listen to the teen's feelings without judgment, and without insisting that their standards are the only ones that are important. If they can be supportive on a daily basis, they become a resource equally as important to recovery as professional help.

CHANGING THE PATTERN

PARENTS

❦   If your cultural background is different from that of the dominant culture, take seriously the impact this has on your children's feelings about their bodies and self-esteem. They may be caught in a cross-current that is very confusing.

❦   Open your heart to hear your daughter's struggle with her body image. Her feelings are real and need to be heard.

❦   Realize that your daughter's situation may require professional counseling and the help of antidepressant medication. Depression is a very real medical condition and often accompanies body concerns and the onset of an eating disorder.

❧ If your daughter needs professional help, do not take it personally. This doesn't mean that you are not a good parent. It is not uncommon for a girl to need outside counsel in addition to parental love and support.

❧ When helping her choose a therapist, consider that she may need a counselor who understands your culture or has a similar cultural background.

❧ Remember: Your role is vital. Nothing can replace the importance of a family's love and understanding.

TEENS

❧ Remember: Although it is hard to straddle two cultures, you are in a unique position to understand both. That understanding may help you find a solution.

❧ If you are having difficulty balancing both parts of your bicultural experience, seek a trusted adult who can understand both cultural experiences.

❧ Don't back down. Your feelings are legitimate and need to be shared with your family. Take the chance to tell them your dilemma.

❧ If your parents don't understand your need for professional help, seek a school counselor, coach, or teacher to hear your concerns and help to explain them to your parents.

❧ Don't use fashion magazines as an indicator of what healthy bodies look like. The pictures you see are almost always airbrushed to make models look unnaturally thin.

SUPPLEMENTARY RESOURCES

FOR PARENTS AND TEENS
Bilingual/Bicultural Family Network
www.biculturalfamily.org

A network of families around the world who are raising their children bilingually and/or biculturally providing support and resources to one another

Conclusion

PERFECTING THE ART OF BALANCE

*Feelings of worth can flourish only in an atmosphere where
individual differences are appreciated, mistakes are tolerated,
communication is open, and rules are flexible—the kind of
atmosphere that is found in a nurturing family.*

—Virginia Satir

The purpose of *Conquering Eating Disorders* is to educate and bring awareness to the various disguises under which eating disorders can invade the lives of an entire family. It is our sincere hope that parents and teens, after reading this book, feel better equipped with the tools they need to enable them to fight against this insidious disorder. Parents and teens both must recognize the importance of working together and sharing in the balance of responsibility for recovery. We hope the following advice will serve your family well.

FOR PARENTS:

Your role in recovery is about giving and giving and more giving—giving of your time, your energy, and especially of your love. If your attitude is restricting, your teen will continue to restrict. If your approach is giving, they may learn to give to themselves.

This role may sometimes feel like the ultimate balancing act. Teens will remind you of that with their sometimes unpredictable—and sometimes negative—reactions to your sincere attempts to be authentic and to give of yourself. We hope that the following advice will help you keep your equilibrium as you step up to the challenge.

First of all, remember that you have not caused the eating disorder, nor can you provide the solution. Therefore, it is unfair to blame yourself. At the same time, however, it is important to examine ways that you yourself need to change in order to support your child's recovery. The balance here is to take responsibility for this self-examination—making small-course corrections in your patterns—while at the same time permitting your teen to be fully responsible for his or her own role in healing. Without blaming yourself, you can examine such tendencies as being overprotective, being afraid of feelings (your teen's or your own), having overly valued attitudes about food and weight, or not making enough one-on-one time with your teen.

Self-examination must be honest without turning into self-blame. If you blame yourself or start to feel defensive, you may become so self-absorbed that you miss out on the learning that could make a big difference in your teen's healing. By blaming yourself, you are also giving your teen permission to blame you, and in a way, you're saying that you have all the power. Actually, your teen needs the power. The most helpful message you can give your child is that you have confidence that he or she can take the necessary steps toward recovery, and that you will be there for support. In addition, you can acknowledge that you are willing to make the necessary changes in yourself, or in your role in the family dynamics. These efforts on your part bring your teenager's derailed development back on course, paving the way to a normal life again.

Remember that you cannot be her therapist and shouldn't try to play that role. She may need a professional and a group of recovering peers to give her assistance and perspective, and to help her discover the hidden messages underneath her troublesome symptoms. This decoding process is a way of looking at the purposes the eating disorder has been serving, and how it was mistakenly perceived as saving your teen or your family from even deeper pain. Though misdirected, this effort to rescue oneself or one's family needs to be honored and acknowledged, and then faced head-on.

The recovery process is demanding because it requires getting at the hidden messages underlying the symptoms. Although it's difficult and requires new behaviors and attitudes on both your parts, it can also be transforming. Developing a new identity, and discovering new possibilities and interests, can result in growth for the teen that would never have occurred without having gone through the eating disorder. Many clients report that recovery made them stronger and more self-defined. And in fact, the eating disorder—which is, in essence, a cry for help—can be the teen's first step on the road to a stronger recognition of who she is, how she feels, and what she wants to become. Just as scar tissue is stronger than regular tissue, a young person can gain resilience through recovery—resilience that will fortify her and increase her appreciation for life's joys and lessons.

Another challenging balancing act is how to be supportive and listen without being overprotective and intrusive. After all, you are needed as a sounding board, not as a problem manager. But knowing when to step in and when to back off can be tricky. Stepping in when it's not needed robs your teen of autonomy. Keeping your distance when she is giving signals that she *does* need you can be hurtful. Too much help can be suffocating; too little may feel like an abandonment.

You may need your teen's coaching to help you reach this balance. You *will* make mistakes and must trust your teen to tell you how much involvement is enough. Above all, try to be honest with every word and action. Remember the importance of little things such as a smile, a touch, a listening ear, or even the offer of a glass of water.

Focusing on your *own* needs is also important. You must keep a life of your own and not let her eating disorder destroy your separate existence. Ask any parent with an eating-disordered teen, and he or she will warn you about the danger of losing yourself in your child's problem. The effective balance here is caring for yourself and honoring your own time and activities while being sensitive to her cries for help. Don't let the talons of the eating disorder threaten to pierce your sense of self—or hers. She needs your strength and individuality to bolster her healing and give her hope that she can recover.

Being knowledgeable about eating disorders will help you keep a healthy distance and maintain good boundaries, but herein lies another paradox. Overeducating yourself about what to expect may keep you from listening to your teen's very personal and individual story, and may cause you to stereotype the problem. Your teen is unique and will need you to understand how her experience may differ from the textbook version.

Finally, just as your teen needs to share feelings and experiences, so do you. Your honest self-disclosure of thoughts and emotions is very important. If you want your child to grasp reality instead of being in denial, you must be honest about the effects the eating disorder is having on you and others in the family. On the other hand, you don't want to burden your teen with all of your problems. This is definitely another balancing act for you. *Share* your feelings, but don't give her the burden of *fixing* your problem on top of her own. Her efforts need to be focused on her own recovery.

We realize that maintaining this balance is a tall order. Remember that, above all, you do not have to be perfect. Especially if your teen has a strong streak of perfectionism, be sure to take it easy, and allow for mistakes: You don't want to be the model of something your child is already struggling with. Even if your teenager seems to be pushing you away, she will model her behavior after yours. Kids have a way of being loyal to parents even when they seem the most distant.

Sometimes it is a challenge for a parent to convince a son or daughter to go to a therapist. It may help to suggest one session, during which a professional can evaluate whether there is an eating disorder involved. The purpose of that first visit is just evaluation, but it also provides an opportunity for the professional to establish rapport and paves the way for ongoing therapy, if it is needed. This approach can be less intimidating than an initial conversation about rushing into therapy. Occasionally, a parent is overreacting, and an astute therapist can help make that determination.

We wish new growth for you and your teenager as you extend your love and support to each other. Remember that your contribution to your child's recovery is in sharing your honesty and uniqueness with her through every act of love and kindness, great and small.

FOR TEENS:

Your role in your own recovery goes without saying. Your parents cannot fix this problem for you, but their support and personal changes are vital to your becoming whole. This recovery journey may feel lonely and frightening. The basic problems that you have covered up with your disordered eating may reappear after you give it up. You may at first feel more depressed as you face issues that you felt you couldn't face before, when you resorted to an unhealthy relationship with food and disconnected from your body.

An eating disorder can feel as if it's taken on a personality of its own. This can actually be a helpful way to look at the eating disorder—as something separate from yourself. You may feel that it helped you through a tough period in your journey toward adulthood. But as you gain more understanding of the reasons it seemed necessary at the time, you will see that *now* is the time to break free and sever yourself from this destructive and dependent relationship.

As you face the intense feelings that lie under the eating disorder, you will see that you *can* deal with emotions and master situations that you thought were insurmountable. You will become a better problem-solver and will lose your phobia about eating normally. You will replace this preoccupation with food and weight with new coping skills and new interests. Thinking continually about food, planning binges, recovering from purging, and worrying about your body takes a great deal of time. Now you will have time for the joys in life: new relationships, new passions, and new goals for the future. You will begin to realize how much more important you are on the inside than on the outside. You will begin to experience yourself as a complex and wonderful person with feelings you didn't know you had, with dreams for the future, and with contributions you can make to the world through your own unique gifts. Life will take on new texture and new excitement as you leave behind the obsession with food, your body, and your appearance and begin to focus on making a difference in the world and in the lives of those around you.

You are not alone on this journey of recovery. Hopefully, this book has given your parents new ideas about how to support you, and how to change what they need to change in themselves. If you have opened your heart to them and have dared to be honest, they will know you better and will know more about what you need and how you feel. They cannot read your mind and can only help you when you help them to understand.

You may also have professionals available to help you if you need them. In fact, you may have a team around you to fine-tune your recovery process. This team could include a medical doctor, a therapist, a dietitian, and a supportive group of others who are in the recovery process with you.

We wish you success in your journey. We trust that you will love your body again and will develop a healthy relationship with food as you transform it from an enemy into a friend. Above all, we believe that you can become whole and find joy within yourself and with others. Remember that there is only *one* of you: No one who has ever lived has been exactly like you, and no one in the future will ever be you. You are unique and precious, just as you are. We salute you as you face the future with courage and determination. Treasure yourself, love others, and freely give your gifts to the world.

Appendix

TOOLS FOR FAMILIES

FAMILY MEALS ARE POWERFUL

Sitting down to eat dinner as a family almost seems countercultural in today's fast-paced world. Yet there is increasing evidence that family meals might do more for children's well-being and sense of accomplishment than any sports program or extracurricular activity. It is certainly one of the few times in modern society that families get together and talk, face to face—making mealtime an excellent opportunity to build relationships.

According to a University of Minnesota survey for Project EAT[1], teens who eat dinner with their families tend to have higher grade-point averages and are more well adjusted. They are less likely to feel depressed or suicidal, smoke cigarettes, use alcohol, or abuse substances. In addition, children who eat regular meals with their families eat more healthfully—incorporating more fruits, vegetables, and calcium-rich foods, and fewer soft drinks. This may also put them at a lower risk for developing an eating disorder.

TIPS ON MAXIMIZING THE MEALTIME

EXPERIENCE

❧ Parents can model good eating habits and show their children what a "normal" meal looks like by including a variety of foods and tastes. They can set a good example by eating slowly and enjoying the meal.

❧ Avoid making anyone eat everything on his or her plate. Rather, honor each individual's hunger and fullness— letting each person decide when he or she is finished.

❧ Meals should have a starting and a stopping point so that teens don't feel "stuck at the table" and unable to get on with their lives. An average meal should last about a half-hour to an hour.

❧ Mealtime is a time to involve the kids in planning, cooking, serving, and cleanup. The more involved they are, the more likely they are to make meals a priority. This is a great opportunity for them to learn how to prepare a healthy meal—a skill that will come in handy when they head out on their own.

❧ Storytelling, playing word games, and including everyone in the conversation can build confidence. The quality of the conversation can actually help children become better readers—exposed to new words, they can increase their vocabularies.

❧ If there's a time crunch, get takeout, go to a restaurant, or, instead of dinner, try to eat breakfast or lunch as a family. This sends the message to your kids that you value your time together.

❧ Conflicts or difficult discussions have no place at the family dinner table. Make mealtime a pleasant experience—something you all look forward to at the end of a busy day.

1. *N. I. Larsen, D. Neuwork-Szetainer, P. J. Hannan, and M. Story, "Family Meals during Adolescence Are Associated with Higher Diet Quality and Healthful Meal Patterns during Young Adulthood," Journal of the American Dietetic Association 107 (2007): 1502–10.*

TOOLS FOR FAMILIES

FAMILY MEETINGS ENHANCE
GOOD COMMUNICATION

Effective communication is the hallmark of successful families. But as they struggle to keep up with the demands of work, school, and extracurricular activities, today's busy family members often find themselves running in opposite directions. As a result, there is little time to talk, resolve problems, or even have fun with one another.

Family meetings can be a way to rectify that. They can be used to deal with a variety of issues, including discussing problems, planning activities and vacations, talking about chores, sharing positive experiences, and having fun.

A family meeting is a prearranged or structured time that a family has agreed to spend together to talk about what is going on in their lives. At first, it's best to keep family meetings short— about fifteen to twenty minutes. As family members get more comfortable with sharing and discussing issues, the meeting times can be lengthened.

TIPS TO GET STARTED

✎   Hold family meetings on a regular basis. Once a week works well for most families, but twice a month may work better for others. The benefit of regularly scheduled meetings is that they open lines of communication and help parents and teens work together to problem-solve within a group.

✎   Encourage all family members to attend, but don't force the issue. When those who choose not to attend see that everyone else is enjoying the meeting, or that they are missing out on decision-making, they will most likely want to join in.

✎   Make sure everyone has a chance to express their views. Share joys and achievements, as well as problems and concerns. Avoid focusing only on the negative, so that family members will stay interested and want to attend.

✎   Strive for consensus when decisions are being made, making sure each person feels heard. However, there will be times when everyone cannot agree. In these instances, a popular vote can be taken.

❧ Plan some fun activities for the whole family—taking into account the different age ranges of your children. Perhaps a picnic in the park, a hike, a trip to the ice-cream parlor, or a board game would be a good idea. Make sure everyone has a voice, or that you take turns doing something each member of the family would enjoy.

TOOLS FOR FAMILIES

THE GIFT OF FORGIVENESS

In the process of recovering from an eating disorder, parents and teens may express feelings that indicate they have been hurt by another family member, often inadvertently. Sharing experiences and feelings that have been bottled up usually helps the process of recovery, because honesty cleanses and heals. In the process, a parent often learns about an action or words that have cut deeply, or that have been misinterpreted. In addition, teens suffering from the eating disorder sometimes hurt parents or siblings by sneaking food, hiding purging behavior, isolating themselves, or withholding information that indicates a serious medical problem.

Learning that something we have done has been hurtful or even devastating to another is not easy, especially when our intention was not to cause harm or negative feelings. There can be a tendency to nurse wounds in silence or not acknowledge the hurt caused to another. However, to move beyond hurt or misunderstanding, forgiveness may be important to ask for and receive. There is power in telling someone that you did not mean to cause pain, and asking that person for forgiveness. It is not unusual to hear a teen say, "She never told me she was sorry, even after I explained that her actions made me feel worse about myself." Conversely, when a parent asks a teen for forgiveness for saying something that hurt, or when a teen apologizes for her secretiveness and asks a parent to forgive her, the result can heal a wound that could otherwise lie dormant and undermine the relationship.

POINTS TO KEEP IN MIND ABOUT FORGIVENESS

⮞ Remember that asking for forgiveness is a strength, not a weakness.

⮞ Saying "I'm sorry" takes just a minute but can alleviate years of distress and hurt.

⮞ Asking for forgiveness does not always mean you were at fault—but it does mean you are sorry that you caused hurt or pain, even if you had been previously unaware of the reaction.

⮞ Closing the loop by telling a family member that you *do* forgive him or her is a gift of love that is worth its weight in gold. Not only does it bring relief to the person you forgive, but it keeps you from holding on to bitterness and anger.

✍   Even if you apologize and feel regret for the pain you have caused, you cannot force another to forgive you when you have caused hurt. That does not mean your apology and regret are in vain, however. It is healing to apologize.

✍   Even if the person who has hurt you does not ask for forgiveness, you can still forgive and will benefit by letting go of resentment.

TOOLS FOR FAMILIES

THE IMPORTANCE OF
COMMUNICATING WITH "I" MESSAGES

Expressing feelings directly is an important part of effective communication and is key to creating a healing environment within a family. When you need to tell family members that you are upset about something they have said or done, it is human nature to say "*You* always tell me that I am wrong," or "*You* don't understand my feelings."

The word "you" can sound accusatory and can put others on the defensive. Rather than expressing an objection with a blaming word such as "you," it is easier for others to take feedback when you own your feelings, using an "I" message to explain how you are reacting to something they did or said.

An "I" message is a statement you make to another that first describes a situation, then explains a behavior that the other person demonstrated and, most important, conveys the impact that behavior had on you. That impact is usually a feeling word (scared, angry, sad, etc.). For example, when a parent is concerned that her daughter is restricting her eating too much, the parent can be tempted to say, "*You* are going to get sick if you eat only salads." Instead, the mom or dad might say, "Last night, when I noticed that all you ate at dinner was salad, I was really frightened."

Using an "I" message does not necessarily mean that the response will always be positive, but you are much less apt to get a defensive response.

TIPS FOR DEALING WITH CONFLICT

☙ Instead of conveying blame with a "you" message, use an "I" message.

☙ Include the situation, the other person's behavior, and your emotional reaction.

☙ Use a non-blaming, caring tone of voice, even when expressing anger.

SUPPLEMENTARY READING AND
ADDITIONAL RESOURCES

GENERAL SUPPLEMENTARY READING

FOR MOTHERS

The Body Myth: Adult Women and the Pressure to Be Perfect, by Margo Maine and Joe Kelly

I Am Beautiful: A Celebration of Women in Their Own Words, by Woody Winfree and Dana Carpenter

Mom, I Feel Fat!: Becoming Your Daughter's Ally in Developing a Healthy Body Image, by Sharon A. Hersh

FOR MOTHERS AND FATHERS

Afraid to Eat, by Frances M. Berg

Food, Fun n' Fitness: Designing Healthy Lifestyles for Our Children, by Mary C. Friesz

How to Get Your Kid to Eat . . . But Not Too Much: From Birth to Adolescence, by Ellyn Satter

"I'm, Like, SO Fat": Helping Your Teen Make Healthy Choices about Eating and Exercise in a Weight-Obsessed World, by Dianne Neumark-Sztainer

Intuitive Eating: A Revolutionary Program That Works, by Evelyn Tribole and Elyse Resch

Reviving Ophelia: Saving the Selves of Adolescent Girls, by Mary Pipher

The Rules of Normal Eating: A Commonsense Approach for Dieters, Overeaters, Undereaters, Emotional Eaters, and Everyone in Between, by Karen R. Koenig

When to Worry: How to Tell If Your Teen Needs Help, and What to Do about It, by Lisa Boesky

FOR PARENTS OF YOUNG MEN

Making Weight: Healing Men's Conflicts with Food, Weight, Shape & Appearance, by Arnold Anderson, Leigh Cohn, and Thomas Holbrook

FOR TEENS

Body Talk: The Straight Facts on Fitness, Nutrition & Feeling Great about Yourself, by Ann Douglas and Julie Douglas

A Look in the Mirror: Freeing Yourself from the Body Image Blues, by Valerie Rainon McManus

Over It: A Teen's Guide to Getting Beyond Obsessions with Food and Weight, by Carol Emery Normandi and Lauralee Roark

We Are More Than Beautiful: 46 Real Teen Girls Speak Out about Beauty, Happiness, Love and Life, edited by Woody Winfree

What's Eating You?: A Workbook for Teens with Anorexia, Bulimia and Other Eating Disorders, by Tammy Nelson

FOR PARENTS AND TEENS

Life without ED: How One Woman Declared Independence from Her Eating Disorder and How You Can Too, by Jenni Schaefer, with Thom Rutledge

Susie Orbach on Eating: Change Your Eating, Change Your Life, by Susie Orbach

SUPPLEMENTARY READING FOR SPECIFIC SCENARIOS

These books are also listed at the end of their respective chapters.

SCENARIO 1: LOST IN THE FOG

FOR PARENTS

Feeling Good, by David Burns

Mind over Mood: Change How You Feel by Changing the Way You Think, by Dennis Greenberger and Christine Padesky

Reinventing Your Life, by Jeffrey E. Young

Thoughts and Feelings: Taking Control of Your Moods and Your Life, by Matthew McKay, Martha Davis, and Patrick Fanning

Parenting Well When You're Depressed: A Complete Resource for Maintaining a Healthy Family, by Alexis D. Henry, Jonathan C. Clayfield, Susan M. Phillips, and Joanne Nicholson

SCENARIO 6: HIDING OUT WITH THE SKELETONS

FOR PARENTS

When Your Child Is Cutting: A Parent's Guide to Helping Children Overcome Self-Injury, by Merry E. McVey-Woble, PhD, Sony Khemlani-Patel, PhD, and Fugen Neziroglu, PhD

FOR TEENS

For Teenagers Living with a Parent Who Abuses Alcohol/Drugs, by Edith Lynn Hornik-Beer

Also, for more information for teens with a parent addicted to alcohol, contact Al-Anon/Alateen: www.al-anon.alateen.org, 1-800-4AL-ANON (1-800-425-2666)

SCENARIO 8: SO LITTLE TIME

FOR PARENTS

The Over-Scheduled Child: Avoiding the Hyper-Parenting Trap, by Alvin Rosenfield and Nicole Wise

SCENARIO 10: A FINAL FAREWELL

FOR TEENS

The Grieving Teen: A Guide for Teenagers and Their Friends, by Helen Fitzgerald

Straight Talk about Death for Teenagers: How to Cope with Losing Someone You Love, by Earl A. Grollman

SCENARIO 12: IN CONTROL

FOR PARENTS AND TEENS

Freeing out Families from Perfectionism, by Thomas S. Greenspon

Never Good Enough: How to Use Perfectionism to Your Advantage Without Letting It Ruin Your Life, by Monica Ramirez Basco

Perfectionism: What's Bad about Being Too Good, by M. Adderholdt and Jan Goldberg

Rewind, Replay, Repeat, by Jeff Bell

When Perfect Isn't Good Enough: Strategies for Coping with Perfectionism, by Marten M. Antony and Richard Swinson

SCENARIO 14: THE RUNNER'S HIGH

FOR PARENTS AND TEENS

The Exercise Balance: What's Too Much, What's Too Little and What's Just Right for You!, by Pauline Powers and Ron Thompson

Nancy Clark's Sports Nutrition Guidebook, 3rd ed., by Nancy Clark

SCENARIO 16: LENGTHENING THE LEASH

FOR PARENTS

Father Hunger: Fathers, Daughters, and the Pursuit of Thinness, by Margo Maine

FOR TEENS

National Sexual Assault Hotline (totally confidential): 1-800-656-HOPE (4673)

RAINN (Rape, Abuse & Incest National Network)
www.rainn.org
America's largest anti–sexual assault organization

Teen Help
www.teenhelp.com
Information for teens, parents, and other adults on issues such as eating disorders, pregnancy, sexual abuse, suicide, depression, and stress

SCENARIO 22: A NEW KIND OF FAMILY

FOR PARENTS

Growing Up with Divorce: Helping Your Child Avoid Immediate and Later Emotional Problems, by Neil Kalter

SCENARIO 24: TWO WORLDS COLLIDE

FOR FOR PARENTS AND TEENS

Bilingual/Bicultural Family Network

www.biculturalfamily.org

A network of families around the world who are raising their children bilingually and/or biculturally providing support and resources to one another

OTHER ORGANIZATIONS AND RESOURCES

Dove's Campaign for Real Beauty:

www.campaignforrealbeauty.com

An excellent resource on body image for moms, mentors, and girls

National Sexual Assault Hotline (totally confidential):
1-800-656-HOPE (4673)

Something Fishy
www.somethingfishy.org

ACKNOWLEDGMENTS

We are very grateful to our clients and their parents, whose stories and struggles inspired us to write this book. We would also like to thank those clients whose enthusiastic response to our initial questionnaire convinced us that a book such as this could be a valuable tool.

To our husbands, Steve and John, and all our kids: a huge thank you for your love, encouragement, valuable insights, creativity, reality checks, meals, humor, and computer smarts.

To Don Schmitz and Gus Lee, fellow authors, and other friends who read the initial manuscript: We appreciate your valuable feedback and helpful remarks.

To Anita Anthony-Huebert: a heartfelt thank you for your excellent editing and enthusiasm for our book. Without Anita, who believed in our dream, our book may never have reached our publisher.

To Jim Lockhart and Melinda Beck: We are so grateful for your legal expertise.

To John Lockhart and Phil Cooper, for their unwavering support, as well as their marketing ideas and suggestions: our sincere thanks.

To Donna Guthrie, author and friend, and to all our friends and family, both professional and personal, whose love and support made this journey worthwhile.

To Wendy Taylor, our editor, for her professionalism, willingness to listen when things got tough, and vision for our book, as well as for her ability to keep us on task: We are extremely grateful.

ABOUT THE AUTHORS

SUE COOPER, PHD

As a licensed psychologist, Sue has specialized in the treatment of eating disorders for more than two decades. She received her Bachelor of Arts degree in English from Dickinson College in Carlisle, Pennsylvania; her Master of Arts degree in counseling psychology from Chapman University in Orange, California; and her PhD in 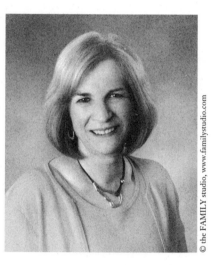 counseling psychology from the University of Denver. She has presented at numerous conferences—international, national, and regional—on the subject of eating-disorder treatment. In addition to her work with eating-disordered clients and their families, Sue is vice president emerita and a core faculty member at the University of the Rockies in Colorado Springs. She is also a feedback coach at the Center for Creative Leadership. She hopes that this book will encourage honest communication and healing conversations between teens and their parents and provide tools to help derail the eating disorders with which these families struggle.

ABOUT THE AUTHORS

PEGGY NORTON, RD

Peggy has worked in the field of dietetics for more than thirty years. She received her Bachelor of Science Degree at Clarke College in Dubuque, Iowa, and completed her Dietetic Internship at Fitzsimmons Army Medical Center in Denver, Colorado. During her military career she worked both as a Staff Dietitian and as an Outpatient Nutrition Counselor at Fitzsimmons. She went on to become the Chief of Clinical Dietetics at Fort Carson Army Hospital in Colorado Springs. In 1980 Peggy was hired by Colorado Surgical Associates to develop and implement the nutrition support for their Gastric Bypass Program and Follow-up Care Plan at Penrose Hospital. After ten years in this position, she opened her private practice and began specializing in eating disorders, working as a team member with therapists. Additionally, Peggy has led groups for eating-disordered clients and overweight individuals. She has been an equine facilitator, partnering with a therapist to develop a specialized program using horse therapy for the

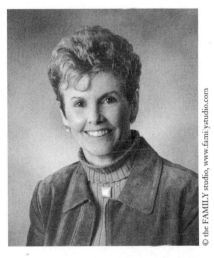

© the FAMILY studio, www.familystudio.com

treatment of eating disorders. This is Peggy's first book. It was born of her desire to reach teenagers and their families—to bring more awareness and understanding of the devastating consequences of eating disorders and to offer hope and healing through the power of telling stories.

INDEX

NOTES

NOTES

NOTES

NOTES

NOTES

NOTES

NOTES

NOTES

NOTES

SELECTED TITLES FROM SEAL PRESS

For more than thirty years, Seal Press has published groundbreaking books. By women. For women. Visit our website at www.sealpress.com.

Body Outlaws: Rewriting the Rules of Beauty and Body Image, edited by Ophira Edut, foreword by Rebecca Walker. $15.95, 1-58005-108-1. Filled with honesty and humor, this groundbreaking anthology offers stories by women who have chosen to ignore, subvert, or redefine the dominant beauty standard in order to feel at home in their bodies.

Reclaiming Our Daughters: What Parenting a Pre-Teen Taught Me About Real Girls, by Karen Stabiner. $14.95, 1-58005-213-9. Offers a message of hope and optimism to the parents of adolescent and preadolescent girls.

I Wanna Be Sedated: 30 Writers on Parenting Teenagers, edited by Faith Conlon and Gail Hudson. $15.95, 1-58005-127-8. With hilarious and heartfelt essays, this anthology will reassure parents of teenagers that they are not alone.

The Bigger, The Better, The Tighter the Sweater: 21 Funny Women on Beauty, Body Image, and Other Hazards of Being Female, edited by Samantha Schoech and Lisa Taggart. $14.95, 1-58005-210-X. A refreshingly honest and funny collection of essays on how women view their bodies.

About Face: Women Write about What They See When They Look in the Mirror, edited by Anne Burt and Christina Baker Kline. $15.95, 1-58005-246-0. 25 women writers candidly examine their own faces—and each face has a story to tell.

Women Who Eat, edited by Leslie Miller. $15.95, 1-58005-092-1. Women both in and out of the culinary profession share their stories about the many ways food shapes and enhances their lives.